The
Pediatric Visit
Gastroenterology

Editors

Leonard G. Feld, MD, PhD, MMM, FAAP
John D. Mahan, MD, FAAP

American Academy of Pediatrics
DEDICATED TO THE HEALTH OF ALL CHILDREN®

American Academy of Pediatrics Publishing Staff

Mary Lou White, *Chief Product and Services Officer/SVP, Membership, Marketing, Publishing*

Mark Grimes, *Vice President, Publishing*

Carrie Peters, *Editor, Professional/Clinical Publishing*

Theresa Wiener, *Production Manager, Clinical and Professional Publications*

Peg Mulcahy, *Manager, Art Direction and Production*

Linda Smessaert, MSIMC, *Senior Marketing Manager, Professional Resources*

Mary Louise Carr, MBA, *Marketing Manager, Clinical Publications*

Published by the American Academy of Pediatrics

345 Park Blvd

Itasca, IL 60143

Telephone: 630/626-6000

Facsimile: 847/434-8000

www.aap.org

The American Academy of Pediatrics is an organization of 67,000 primary care pediatricians, pediatric medical subspecialists, and pediatric surgical specialists dedicated to the health, safety, and well-being of infants, children, adolescents, and young adults.

The recommendations in this publication do not indicate an exclusive course of treatment or serve as a standard of medical care. Variations, taking into account individual circumstances, may be appropriate.

Statements and opinions expressed are those of the authors and not necessarily those of the American Academy of Pediatrics.

Products are mentioned for informational purposes only. Inclusion in this publication does not imply endorsement by the American Academy of Pediatrics.

The publishers have made every effort to trace the copyright holders for borrowed materials. If they have inadvertently overlooked any, they will be pleased to make the necessary arrangements at the first opportunity.

This publication has been developed by the American Academy of Pediatrics. The contributors are expert authorities in the field of pediatrics. No commercial involvement of any kind has been solicited or accepted in development of the content of this publication. Disclosures: Dr Mahan has indicated relationships with Relypsa and Vifor; Dr Rao has indicated a relationship with GlaxoSmithKline; Dr Rosh has indicated relationships with AbbVie, Janssen, and Pfizer.

Every effort has been made to ensure that the drug selection and dosages set forth in this text are in accordance with the current recommendations and practice at the time of publication. It is the responsibility of the health care professional to check the package insert of each drug for any change in indications or dosage and for added warnings and precautions.

Every effort is made to keep *The Pediatric Visit: Gastroenterology* consistent with the most recent advice and information available from the American Academy of Pediatrics.

Special discounts are available for bulk purchases of this publication. Email Special Sales at aapsales@aap.org for more information.

© 2019 American Academy of Pediatrics

Printed in the United States of America

9-421/0519   1 2 3 4 5 6 7 8 9 10

MA0918

ISBN: 978-1-61002-308-5

eBook: 978-1-61002-309-2

Cover design by Linda Diamond

Book design by Peg Mulcahy

Library of Congress Control Number: 2018955228

CONTRIBUTORS

Neetu Bali, MD, MPH
Assistant Professor of Pediatrics
Division of Gastroenterology,
  Hepatology and Nutrition
Nationwide Children's Hospital
Columbus, OH

Ricardo A. Caicedo, MD, FAAP
Associate Professor of Pediatrics
Division of Gastroenterology, Hepatology
  and Nutrition
Levine Children's Hospital
Charlotte, NC

Lay Har Cheng, MD, MSPH
Division of Gastroenterology, Hepatology
  and Nutrition
Levine Children's Hospital
Charlotte, NC

Carmen Cuffari, MD
Associate Professor of Pediatrics
The Johns Hopkins University School
  of Medicine
Baltimore, MD

James F. Daniel, MD
Endowed Chair in Liver Care
Professor of Pediatrics
Children's Mercy Hospital
University of Missouri Kansas City
Kansas City, MO

Jason E. Dranove, MD
Division of Gastroenterology, Hepatology
  and Nutrition
Levine Children's Hospital
Charlotte, NC

Patricia Eaton, DO, FAAP
Attending Physician, Pediatric Emergency
  Medicine
Arnold Palmer Hospital for Children
Orlando, FL

Ryan T. Fischer, MD, FAAP
Associate Professor of Pediatrics
Division of Gastroenterology
Chief, Section of Hepatology and Liver
  Transplant Medicine
Children's Mercy Hospital
Kansas City, MO

Maya Gharfeh, MD, MPH
Allergy and Asthma Care of Waco
Waco, TX

Vani V. Gopalareddy, MD
Associate Professor of Pediatrics
Director, Hepatology and Liver
  Transplantation
Levine Children's Hospital
Charlotte, NC

Karl Horvath, MD, PhD
Clinical Professor of Pediatrics
The Florida State University of College
  of Medicine
Director, Pediatric Gastroenterology
  Training Program
Center for Pediatric Digestive Health
  and Nutrition
Arnold Palmer Hospital for Children
Orlando, FL

Peter L. Lu, MD, MS
Assistant Professor of Pediatrics
Department of Pediatrics
Division of Gastroenterology,
  Hepatology and Nutrition
Nationwide Children's Hospital/The Ohio
  State University College of Medicine
Columbus, OH

Hayat Mousa, MD
Professor of Pediatrics
University of California at San Diego
San Diego, CA

Samuel Nurko, MD, MPH
Director, Center for Motility and
    Functional Gastrointestinal Disorders
Boston Children's Hospital
Boston, MA

John M. Olsson, MD, CPE, FAAP
Professor of Pediatrics
Division of General Pediatrics
University of Virginia School of Medicine
Charlottesville, VA

J. Duncan Phillips, MD, FACS, FAAP
Surgeon-in-Chief
WakeMed Children's Hospital
Raleigh, NC

Victor M. Piñeiro, MD, AGAF
Medial Director, Division of
    Gastroenterology, Hepatology
    and Nutrition
Levine Children's Hospital
Charlotte, NC

Meenakshi Rao, MD, PhD
Division of Gastroenterology, Hepatology
    and Nutrition
Boston Children's Hospital
Harvard Medical School
Boston, MA

Joel Rosh, MD, FACG, AGAF, FAAP
Professor of Pediatrics
Icahn School of Medicine at Mount Sinai
New York, NY
Director, Pediatric Gastroenterology
Vice Chairman, Clinical Development and
    Research Affairs
Goryeb Children's Hospital/Atlantic
    Children's Health
Morristown, NJ

Ameesh A. Shah, MD
Division of Gastroenterology, Hepatology
    and Nutrition
Levine Children's Hospital
Charlotte, NC

Jyoti Sinha, MD
Pediatric Gastroenterology
Summit Medical Group
Berkley Heights, NJ

Michael J. Steiner, MD, MPH, FAAP
Pediatrician in Chief, UNC Children's
    Hospital
Vice-Chair, Department of Pediatrics
University of North Carolina
Chapel Hill, NC

John R. Stephens, MD, SFHM
Professor of Internal Medicine and
    Pediatrics
Division of Hospital Medicine
University of North Carolina
Chapel Hill, NC

Toba A. Weinstein, MD
Associate Professor of Pediatrics
Division of Pediatric Gastroenterology
Donald and Barbara Zucker School of
    Medicine at Hofstra/Northwell
Cohen Children's Medical Center
Northwell Health
New Hyde Park, NY

Nader N. Youssef, MD, FACG, FAAP
Digestive Healthcare Center
Hillsborough, NJ

▼▲▼▲▼▲▼▲▼▲▼▲▼▲▼▲ ▼▲▼▲▼▲▼▲▼▲▼▲▼▲▼

We are most appreciative to our families for their long-term support and understanding as we have toiled through this and many other projects.

To our loved ones—Barbara, Kimberly, Mitchell, Greg (LF), and Ann, Chas, Mary, Christian, Emily, Elisa, Erika, Aileen, and Kelsey (JM)

▼▲▼▲▼▲▼▲▼▲▼▲▼▲▼ ▼▲▼▲▼▲▼▲▼▲▼▲▼▲▼

CONTENTS

▼▲▼▲▼▲▼▲▼▲▼▲▼▲▼▲▼   ▼▲▼▲▼▲▼▲▼▲▼▲▼▲▼▲▼

▼▲▼▲▼▲▼▲▼▲▼▲▼▲   ▼▲▼▲▼▲▼▲▼▲▼▲▼▲▼

PREFACE

The practice of pediatrics requires rapid access to evidence-based information to make timely diagnoses and provide accurate treatment for common conditions. This is our deliverable to you in *The Pediatric Visit*, which focuses on major issues in pediatric gastroenterology. Each chapter emphasizes diagnosis and treatment and includes many figures and tables designed to assist pediatric clinicians in delivering the highest quality of care to patients in the most direct way possible.

Understanding medical decision-making is the foundation on which practitioners make the right decisions at the right time for patients. We present evidence-based levels of decision support (as appropriate) in each chapter to provide valuable information about the level of evidence for diagnostic testing and evaluation, as well as for different treatment modalities.

The levels of evidence in this book are adapted from Harris, Helfand, and Woolf[1]—Level I: evidence obtained from at least 1 properly designed randomized controlled trial; Level II-1: evidence obtained from well-designed controlled trials without randomization; Level II-2: evidence obtained from well-designed cohort or case-control analytic studies, preferably from more than 1 center or research group; Level II-3: evidence obtained from multiple time series, with or without the intervention (dramatic results from uncontrolled trials also might be regarded as Level II-3); and Level III: opinions of respected authorities based on clinical experience, descriptive studies, or reports from expert committees.

We truly appreciate the wonderful guidance and assistance from the American Academy of Pediatrics. Our editor, Carrie Peters, was extremely helpful in the development of this key resource.

We hope that you will find this book on pediatric gastroenterology an indispensable resource for the evaluation and management of your patients.

Leonard G. Feld, MD, PhD, MMM, and John D. Mahan, MD

---

[1] Harris RP, Helfand M, Woolf SH, et al. Current methods of the US Preventive Services Task Force: a review of the process. *Am J Prev Med.* 2001;20(3 suppl):21–35

Acute Abdominal Emergencies

J. Duncan Phillips, MD

OVERVIEW

Fortunately, most children never require urgent evaluation for life-threatening abdominal conditions. However, primary care clinicians may occasionally encounter children in the office or clinic with undiagnosed or untreated illnesses that can rapidly progress, leading to morbidity and even death. Although no primary care clinician should be expected to be an expert on abdominal surgical emergencies, familiarity with the most common conditions, as well as reasonable approaches to their evaluation, is expected. Abdominal emergency conditions discussed in this chapter are malrotation/midgut volvulus, pyloric stenosis, intussusception, Meckel diverticulum disease (bleeding, obstruction, diverticulitis), ingested foreign bodies, cholecystitis, ovarian torsion, and ruptured ovarian cysts. Some conditions may require immediate surgical evaluation and treatment (eg, midgut volvulus and ovarian torsion) while others may need more careful evaluation before surgery (eg, pyloric stenosis). Acute appendicitis is the most commonly encountered emergency surgical condition in children (see Chapter 2).

When called to assess children with suspected abdominal surgical situations, the clinician can be guided by the mnemonic REO (**r**esuscitate *then* **e**valuate *then* possibly **o**perate, *in that order*).

MALROTATION/VOLVULUS

Overview/Definitions

Malrotation is a congenital anomaly of midgut rotation in which the entire small intestine can suddenly twist its vascular pedicle, including the superior mesenteric artery (SMA) and superior mesenteric vein (SMV), causing blockage of the gastrointestinal (GI) tract or acute intestinal ischemia. Although a person can be born with malrotation, it is the twisting of the vasculature (midgut volvulus) that typically causes the symptoms and life-threatening condition.

Differential Diagnosis

Acute gastroenteritis (AGE) may be mistaken for volvulus. With AGE, the vomiting may eventually become bilious but typically does not, and diarrhea is common (but quite rare with volvulus). Gastroesophageal reflux disease may affect up to 80% of young children, especially during the first year after birth. Typically, the regurgitation is mild and nonbilious. Other congenital gastrointestinal obstructions, including duodenal atresia/stenosis/web, small intestinal atresia, colonic atresia (quite rare), Hirschsprung disease, and anorectal anomalies (atresia or stenosis), may mimic malrotation/volvulus. Systemic sepsis from other sources often develops the so-called septic ileus pattern, with diffuse gastrointestinal dysmotility and dilation.

Clinical Features/Signs and Symptoms

Malrotation has an incidence of about 1 in 500 live births. Most children with malrotation become symptomatic in the first month after birth (60%) or before age 1 year (80%). Roughly two-thirds of children with malrotation have other congenital anomalies, including omphalocele, gastroschisis, esophageal atresia, duodenal atresia/stenosis/web, biliary atresia, imperforate anus, or congenital diaphragmatic hernia. Children with situs inversus and other "situs" anomalies (such as situs ambiguous, heterotaxy, or heterotaxia) are more likely to have malrotation than children with normal rotation (situs solitus). The most important feature of malrotation (with volvulus) is bilious emesis. True bilious emesis from volvulus is dark green liquid vomit. Green vomit in the neonate indicates malrotation with volvulus until proven otherwise. Although more than 95% of children with midgut volvulus develop vomiting, in up to 20% the vomitus may not be green. Children old enough to speak almost always report having abdominal pain. Less than 20% of children with volvulus develop diarrhea, and it is often bloody mucus or loose stool with blood, which may help differentiate malrotation/volvulus from acute gastroenteritis. Many children develop abdominal distension, but a flat or even scaphoid abdomen does not rule out volvulus. Normal physical examination findings are the hallmark of early midgut volvulus. This is the point at which the patient, and the midgut, are still salvageable. By the time the examination findings become abnormal (with distention and peritoneal signs), the intestine is often already infarcted, or well on its way, and the outcome is often catastrophic.

Evaluation

Evaluation of a child with suspected volvulus takes precedence over almost all other children in one's care. The diagnostic test with the highest accuracy is the upper gastrointestinal (UGI) radiographic series. During this procedure, the physician looks for a corkscrew appearance of the duodenum at the site of the twist. Computed tomography (CT) (with enteral contrast) should be discouraged because it takes time and energy away from an expeditious evaluation. However, if a CT scan has been ordered to help evaluate unexplained abdominal pain and images are available, they typically reveal all small intestine on the right side of the abdomen and the colon on the left side. Ultrasonography may reveal a reversal of the normal relationship of the SMA and SMV, but this finding can be subtle; therefore, this test should be used only in centers with experienced and capable ultrasonographers. A confusing ultrasound test that suggests possible malrotation probably should be followed by an UGI series.

Management

A child with confirmed midgut volvulus requires immediate surgery to untwist the affected intestine. Midgut volvulus may result in intestinal infarction in as little as 2 to 4 hours.

Children with suspected malrotation and volvulus should be transferred immediately to the nearest facility with the ability to perform pediatric surgery. The surgeon should be contacted immediately (even before transfer, if possible). Treatment involves urgent laparotomy (or laparoscopy at some centers) with derotation of the intestine, division of Ladd bands (congenital tissue bands that typically stretch across the duodenum), and rearrangement of the GI tract within the peritoneal cavity. Typically, the patient's appendix ends up in an unusual or abnormal location, so an appendectomy usually is performed to avoid future diagnostic confusion were appendicitis ever to develop.

Long-term Monitoring

Depending on the duration of preoperative symptoms and the tightness of the mesenteric twist, some children suffer from short bowel syndrome, with its associated risks of liver failure due to prolonged total parenteral nutrition and systemic sepsis resulting from infections of central venous catheters.

Some children with rotational anomalies continue to experience symptoms of gastrointestinal dysmotility despite correction of the malrotation, especially in cases of atypical malrotation variants. Some children may continue to have episodic vomiting with or without abdominal pain for many years. Recurrent intestinal obstruction resulting from postoperative adhesions is not uncommon and is a well-recognized outcome in some children following the Ladd procedure for treatment of volvulus.

PYLORIC STENOSIS

Overview/Definition

Pyloric stenosis, also called hypertrophic pyloric stenosis, infantile hypertrophic pyloric stenosis, or congenital hypertrophic pyloric stenosis, is a relatively common disorder of progressive idiopathic thickening of the pyloric muscle, causing worsening partial obstruction of the stomach, with subsequent vomiting of ingested breast milk or formula and gastric secretions. Affected children are typically between the ages of 2 and 6 weeks. Boys are affected 4 to 5 times more frequently than girls, with the most commonly affected child being a firstborn male. Occasionally, there is a history of pyloric stenosis in parents or other relatives. A clear association has been reported between pyloric stenosis and early exposure to erythromycin (between 3 and 13 days after birth) (Evidence Level II-2).

Causes and Differential Diagnosis

The exact cause of pyloric stenosis is unknown. It appears to be an acquired illness, not congenital, but there is a definite familial tendency, with the sons of affected mothers having the highest risk. The differential diagnosis includes gastroesophageal reflux (GER) or gastroesophageal reflux disease (GERD), which may affect up to 80% of infants during the first year after birth. With GER/GERD, the regurgitation typically develops earlier (even within the first few days after birth); it may be less forceful and may not lead to significant dehydration and/or weight loss. Acute gastroenteritis (viral or bacterial) may mimic pyloric stenosis, but the former is typically associated with diarrhea and/or fever. Meningitis or other causes of central nervous system irritation also may mimic pyloric stenosis; in children with such conditions, irritability and vomiting may be the primary manifestations.

Clinical Features

Most infants with pyloric stenosis present with progressively worsening postprandial nonbilious emesis. They typically vomit within several minutes after eating (up to 30 to 60 minutes in some cases). The vomiting may be quite forceful (projectile). With worsening emesis, infants eventually tire and may become dehydrated and lethargic.

Evaluation

Many pediatric surgeons recommend decompressing the air-filled stomach by aspirating it with a small orogastric decompression tube. Infants are then allowed to drink a small amount of glucose water from a bottle, which seems to provide comfort in most cases and allows relaxation of the tensed, contracted abdominal wall musculature. The examiner typically feels the enlarged muscle—about the size and shape of a cocktail olive—in the epigastrium, either in the midline or slightly to the right, and approximately halfway between the umbilicus and the xiphoid. Even in experienced hands, a significant percentage of children will not have the palpable "olive" appreciated; consequently, most children with pyloric stenosis undergo preoperative ultrasonography, the test of choice. It shows a thickened and elongated pyloric channel, often without passage of gastric contents through the pylorus. Upper gastrointestinal radiography can be performed as well. However, radiography entails radiation exposure and typically is performed only when gastroesophageal reflux or other congenital partial obstructions are suspected.

Laboratory assessment often shows hypochloremic or hypokalemic metabolic alkalosis. Approximately one-third of affected infants may have slight jaundice or sclera icterus. Gastrointestinal jaundice is metabolic in origin and resolves quickly after pyloromyotomy in most infants. Therefore, extensive laboratory evaluation or workup typically is not required.

Management

Most children with pyloric stenosis require fluid resuscitation and correction of an electrolyte abnormality. Preoperative resuscitation may take as little as 6 to 8 hours or as long as several days, depending on the degree of electrolyte disturbance. General anesthesia in an infant with significant alkalosis is inadvisable because the drive to breathe at the end of the operation is primarily driven by brainstem chemoreceptors that may be "buffered" by excess base. An easy way to assess alkalosis correction is to monitor serum chloride levels—typically, if they are greater than the mid-90s (in milliequivalents of chloride per liter of blood), the risks are relatively low.

Pyloric stenosis is treated with pyloromyotomy, with longitudinal cutting and spreading of the pyloric muscle fibers, without damage to the underlying submucosa and mucosa. This operation can be performed via laparotomy as an "open" procedure or laparoscopically.

Up to two-thirds of surgically treated children continue to have at least mild emesis, which typically resolves over several days, but may persist for several weeks. True recurrent pyloric stenosis, in which the cut muscle edges reattach, is extremely rare. Gastroesophageal reflux and overfeeding are the 2 most common causes of persistent emesis after pyloromyotomy.

Long-term Monitoring

Long-term follow-up studies of adults who underwent pyloric stenosis surgery in infancy show no obvious abnormalities in foregut function or an increased risk of peptic ulcer disease (Evidence Level II-2).

INTUSSUSCEPTION

Overview/Definitions

Intussusception occurs when a segment of the intestine invaginates (telescopes) into the next (downstream) segment of the intestine. Most intussusceptions in children (80%–90%) are idiopathic, believed to be secondary to thickened Peyer patches of lymphatic tissue in the intestinal wall, which acts as a lead point (intussusceptum). Occasionally, children have an abnormal anatomic structure within the intussusceptum. Common lead points include Meckel diverticula, intestinal polyps, and intestinal tumors such as lymphomas. In adolescents and adults, intussusception is almost always caused by tumors. Intussusception may also occur following rotavirus vaccination. The pathophysiology is likely similar to that of idiopathic intussusception, with enlargement of lymphatic tissue in the wall of the distal ileum.

While idiopathic intussusception occurs most often in children between 5 and 12 months of age, it is not unusual to observe the condition in children aged 2 to 4 years. If diagnosed early, most cases of intussusception can be treated nonoperatively, with barium or air reduction via enema. Persistent uncorrected intussusception can result in intestinal infarction, perforation, systemic sepsis, and death. Intussusception in older children or children with repeated intussusceptions should prompt a workup for a specific lead point such as a diverticulum or polyp.

Differential Diagnosis

Acute gastroenteritis is probably the most common mimic of intussusception because viral or bacterial enteritis occurs so frequently in young children, and the symptoms (vomiting, abdominal pain, possible fever) may be identical to those of early intussusception (before the passage of mucus in the stool). Other causes of intestinal obstruction may resemble intussusception, including incarcerated inguinal hernias, tumors, and internal hernias. It is not unusual for a ruptured appendix to be walled off in the right lower quadrant, causing a kink in the terminal ileum that resembles intussusception.

Clinical Features

When intussusception occurs, with each series of intestinal contractions, there is stretching of the intestinal wall, which causes severe, crampy pain. An infant with intussusception typically has a sudden onset of crying and screaming and pulls the knees up toward the abdomen. When the attack ends after several minutes, the infant may appear healthy and resumes activity. These attacks of colicky pain with pain-free intervals, which can occur every 10 to 30 minutes, are a classic finding with intussusception. They can be quite dramatic and frightening to parents and other caregivers. Other symptoms include vomiting and passage of blood per rectum. However, this triad (vomiting, pain, blood) occurs in less than 20% of cases.

If intussusception is not treated, it may lead to systemic sepsis, with lethargy, mental status changes, hypotension, and even shock.

Evaluation

Although somewhat controversial, most children with suspected intussusception initially undergo a 2-view abdominal radiographic series (kidney, ureter, and bladder [KUB] and upright) (Evidence Level III). The KUB findings may be mildly abnormal, but they are rarely completely diagnostic. Dance sign, the presence of an upper abdominal mass with a paucity or absence of air in the right lower quadrant, may be diagnostic but is rarely seen. The presence of the cecal air shadow in the right lower quadrant does not necessarily rule out intussusception because this can be a normal finding in infants younger than 12 months. Despite the limitations of the KUB, it may allow a rough estimation of the severity of the intestinal obstruction, if present, and a determination of any radiographic evidence of pneumoperitoneum (so-called free air), which points to probable intestinal perforation. Although rare, if pneumoperitoneum is documented, no further radiographic studies usually are obtained; intravenous antibiotics are started to treat peritonitis; and an urgent pediatric surgery consultation is obtained. Because peritonitis usually can be diagnosed by means of a physical examination of the abdomen, some clinicians do not believe that the KUB is necessary before obtaining an ultrasound study or a contrast enema (Evidence Level III).

If pneumoperitoneum is not found, and if the child is in a center with an ultrasonographer with appropriate experience and skill, the next test may be an abdominal ultrasound study. Typically, a so-called target sign would suggest intussusception. The target sign is the cross-sectional appearance of a thickened portion of intestine that has become lodged in the lumen of the more downstream intestine, thus giving the appearance of an archery target. It is important to point out that negative ultrasound study findings do not necessarily rule out intussusception, and a contrast enema study may still be needed (see later in this chapter).

Management

If the ultrasound study confirms intussusception (or it is strongly suspected on clinical grounds), a contrast enema, using air (introduced under pressure) or barium, typically is the next step. A radiologist introduces a small tube into the infant's anus and uses air (with a small squeezable hand pump similar to a blood pressure cuff) or barium (from a small bag, typically elevated above the infant on an intravenous pole) to fill the rectum and colon in a retrograde fashion. The purpose is to confirm the intussusception diagnosis and reduce the intussusception, thus avoiding the need for surgical intervention. Pneumatic reduction, with air, has a higher reported success rate (typically 80% to 90%). Some studies suggest that air reduction may involve a somewhat higher risk of perforation than hydrostatic reduction. If hydrostatic or pneumatic reduction is unsuccessful, or if diffuse peritonitis is present, the child requires urgent surgical treatment.

Following hydrostatic or pneumatic reduction, about 3% of patients experience a recurrence of crampy abdominal pain, usually within 1 to 2 days after the initial reduction. If this occurs, most patients can be returned to the radiology suite for a second reduction.

Long-term Monitoring

Most children with intussusception who are promptly diagnosed and treated respond well, with no long-term sequelae. Survival is higher than 95%. Most deaths occur when patients do not receive medical attention soon enough after the onset of symptoms. Infants who have had intussusception for 48 to 72 hours may become profoundly dehydrated and develop hypotension and shock. They may also develop systemic sepsis from the release of toxic metabolites from an ischemic/infarcted intestine.

Rarely, intussusception recurs within a few days of successful surgical reduction. If that happens, the child typically presents with similar symptoms and may require repeated hydrostatic or pneumatic reduction.

MECKEL DIVERTICULUM

Overview/Definitions

Meckel diverticulum is a congenital full-thickness intestinal outpouching of the distal ileum. It is often referred to as "the organ of 2s" because it is said to be present in roughly 2% of the general population, is typically 2 inches long (depending on the patient's age) and is found roughly 2 feet proximal to the ileocecal junction.

Differential Diagnosis

The differential diagnosis depends on the presenting signs and symptoms. If the patient presents with gastrointestinal bleeding, the differential includes multiple conditions: infectious gastroenteritis/colitis, anal fissure, vascular malformations of the GI tract (such as hemangiomas), inflammatory bowel disease (including ulcerative colitis and Crohn disease), intestinal tumors/polyps, and nonaccidental trauma (sexual abuse/instrumentation). If the child presents with evidence of gastrointestinal obstruction, the differential diagnosis includes adhesive small bowel obstruction (usually secondary to previous intra-abdominal procedures), appendicitis (usually ruptured), malrotation/volvulus, internal hernia (through a congenital mesenteric defect), and incarcerated abdominal wall hernia (inguinal/femoral/umbilical). Finally, if the child presents with Meckel diverticulitis, the differential diagnosis includes infectious gastroenteritis/colitis or appendicitis.

Clinical Features

Bleeding

If a patient develops bleeding because of Meckel diverticulum, it typically produces painless hematochezia. Parents typically note large, brick-red (or purple) bloody stools. Bleeding typically is episodic and stops spontaneously. Black "tarry" stools are less common.

Bleeding may be voluminous, with roughly half of children requiring preoperative blood transfusions. As a result, some children develop pallor, tachycardia, and even shock.

Obstruction

Children with obstruction have waves of crampy abdominal pain, emesis that becomes bilious, decreased stool output, and abdominal distension. The abdominal examination may reveal diffuse tenderness.

Diverticulitis

Diverticulitis may be indistinguishable from acute appendicitis, with lower abdominal pain, tenderness, nausea, vomiting, and fever; however, the location of the pain may be somewhat more medial. With perforation, the pain typically becomes diffuse, with the development of peritonitis.

Evaluation

Bleeding

The most useful test for Meckel diverticulum is usually technetium Tc 99m pertechnetate scintigraphy, which is concentrated in gastric mucosa.

Obstruction

Plain abdominal radiographs (the so-called KUB and upright) should identify children with a small bowel obstruction. The upright film (or cross-table lateral images in children too small or weak to stand) typically show multiple air-fluid levels suggestive of obstruction rather than an adynamic ileus.

Diverticulitis

Tests include a complete blood cell count. Although ultrasonography and CT have been described as helpful, these tests may not be necessary in children with suspected appendicitis (which is often the preoperative diagnosis in children with Meckel diverticulitis).

Management

Symptomatic diverticula should be resected either via a laparotomy as an "open" procedure or with laparoscopic techniques.

Long-term Monitoring

Children are at risk for the usual complications of abdominal surgery, including adhesion formation and intestinal obstruction. Adhesive intestinal obstructions may occur at any time after abdominal surgery (months, years, or even decades later). Fortunately, the risk is low (<5%–15% for most abdominal operations) (Evidence Level II-3). However, children and parents should be warned that bilious (green) emesis and crampy abdominal pain should prompt a visit to the primary care clinician, emergency department, or surgeon.

▼▲▼▲▼▲▼▲▼▲▼▲▼▲▼   ▼▲▼▲▼▲▼▲▼▲▼▲▼▲▼

INGESTED FOREIGN BODIES

Overview/Definitions

Foreign bodies are items not usually associated with normal eating habits, such as coins or other metallic objects. A trichobezoar is a mass composed of ingested hair, which may become tightly packed and compressed. The most common location for a trichobezoar is the stomach, but some patients may have smaller ones in their small intestine.

Coins are the most common ingested foreign body in children. Most ingested foreign bodies, including nails, tacks, and other sharp items, pass spontaneously through the GI tract and do not require endoscopic or surgical removal. Because the narrowest part of the entire GI tract is the cricopharyngeus muscle (the upper esophageal sphincter), unless there is a congenital or acquired stricture more distally or an acquired narrowing because of surgery, most foreign bodies passing this upper sphincter muscle are likely to pass through the rest of the GI tract uneventfully. Exceptions include button batteries, high-power magnets, and sharp objects longer than 3 cm. Ingested batteries (especially watch batteries, or button batteries) may conduct current, resulting in the production of heat and causing full-thickness necrosis of the GI tract. This situation is especially worrisome if the battery is lodged in the esophagus, which can cause erosion into the trachea and even the innominate artery, risking massive exsanguinating hemorrhage, tracheoesophageal fistula, or stricture formation. If the foreign body is lodged in the esophagus, the window for diagnosis and removal may be as short as 4 hours, after which the risk of complication rises dramatically. Therefore, diagnosis and treatment are usually considered an emergency. Trichobezoar formation is almost always a sign of trichotillomania, a serious life-threatening psychiatric disorder that always requires psychological evaluation and treatment to prevent recurrence. Most foreign body ingestions occur out of simple childhood curiosity and do not require formal psychiatric evaluation.

Differential Diagnosis

Children may develop coughing, gagging, choking, and/or retching when foreign bodies, particularly very small items, are lodged in the esophagus or the trachea/airway. Retained barium (or another radiographic contrast material) can appear like a foreign body on a radiograph.

Clinical Features/Signs and Symptoms

Although some foreign body ingestions by young children are witnessed by parents, other caregivers, or other children, this scenario seldom occurs. Foreign body ingestion may be suspected, however, when the child was previously seen with an object that now seems to be missing. Most children cough, choke, or gag at the time of ingestion. In addition, some complain of dysphagia, while others may have constant drooling of saliva. Many children are asymptomatic when they are brought in for an evaluation. Foreign bodies may travel distally and cause intestinal obstruction, which can result in abdominal distension, pain, and eventually bilious emesis. However, this outcome is quite rare. Parents and family members should be reassured to avoid undue alarm.

Evaluation

Plain radiographs are typically sufficient to confirm the diagnosis. If the ingested item is not radiopaque (eg, trichobezoar), a contrast upper GI or an abdominal ultrasound may be needed.

Management

Treatment is based on the location of the lesion and composition of the foreign body.

Esophagus

Coins and other objects at the thoracic inlet typically require endoscopic extraction. Because roughly 25% to 30% of coins lodged in the esophagus pass spontaneously into the stomach after 8 to 16 hours, some advocate for observation and repeated radiographs before endoscopy (Evidence Level II-3). However, button batteries lodged in the esophagus require urgent intervention to prevent full-thickness esophageal injury, with possible perforation or fistula formation into the trachea (see Overview/Definitions).

Stomach

Most metallic foreign bodies in the stomach pass spontaneously, without endoscopic extraction, and the care of most children can be managed on an outpatient basis. Serial radiographs (ie, KUBs) can be obtained every few days to document passage, or parents can inspect the child's stools. Passage may take several weeks or even months. If a button battery is identified in the stomach, hospitalization is recommended for serial radiographs to be obtained every few hours. As long as the battery appears to be moving through the GI tract, continued observation is usually appropriate (Evidence Level II-3). However, if serial radiographs suggest that the battery has stopped moving, an endoscopic or a surgical extraction is necessary to prevent perforation or fistula formation. Trichobezoars usually require laparotomy for gastrostomy and extraction. Some trichobezoars have a long hair extension protruding through the pylorus and down into the duodenum and small bowel (the so-called Rapunzel syndrome).

Small/Large Intestine

Most foreign bodies that have passed through the stomach and moved distally will pass spontaneously. Exceptions include button batteries and items ingested by children with a history of abdominal surgery, who may have adhesions that could impinge on free movement of the intestine within the peritoneal cavity or areas of relative narrowing at the site of anastomoses or strictures. Another recently identified exception is the child who swallows multiple magnets, such as those found in various construction-type toys. Magnets scattered along the GI tract may stick together, causing the formation of multiple enteroenteral fistulae.

Long-term Monitoring

Children with mental health disorders, such as trichophagia, or those with intellectual disability, are at risk for recurrent ingestions.

CHOLECYSTITIS

Overview/Definitions

Cholecystitis is an acute inflammatory process affecting the gallbladder, with complete or partial obstruction of the cystic duct by a gallstone or other sub-stance, that causes bile stasis, gallbladder distension, and possible bacterial overgrowth into the gallbladder wall. Although acalculous cholecystitis may be caused by *Salmonella* or other pathogens, it is quite rare in children and seldom requires surgical intervention. Most cholecystitis in children is secondary to gallstones. Chronic cholecystitis typically refers to chronic mild inflammation of the gallbladder, manifested by transient episodes (gallbladder attacks) triggered by eating greasy or fatty foods. Cholelithiasis is the presence of stones in the gallbladder, while choledocholithiasis refers to gallstones in the common bile duct or common hepatic duct.

Symptomatic cholelithiasis, including cholecystitis, is increasing in fre-quency in children and seems to be more common in the Hispanic population. Children receiving long-term total parenteral nutrition are at increased risk of developing cholelithiasis and are at high risk of developing complications, such as cholecystitis. Some physicians advocate prophylactic cholecystectomy in some children (Evidence Level III). Cholelithiasis is associated with cystic

▼△▼△▼△▼△▼△▼△▼△▼   ▼△▼△▼△▼△▼△▼△▼△▼

fibrosis and hemolytic diseases, including sickle cell anemia, thalassemia, and hereditary spherocytosis. This is caused by the chronic breakdown of hemoglobin, resulting in abnormally high levels of bilirubin and, hence, bilirubin stones. Approximately two-thirds of children with sickle cell anemia develop cholelithiasis by adulthood.

Differential Diagnosis

Gallstone disease can be confused with gallbladder dyskinesia (also called biliary dyskinesia), which is increasingly recognized in children. Biliary dyskinesia is characterized by recurrent attacks of biliary-type symptoms (eg, right upper quadrant abdominal pain, nausea, vomiting, food avoidance). Gallstones are not seen on ultrasound examination. Most patients are female and often between the ages of 12 and 16 years. Workup typically involves a cholecystikinin-stimulated HIDA (hepatobiliary iminodiacetic acid) scan, which shows delayed secretion of isotope by a sluggish gallbladder. These children typically have chronic attacks of pain but do not usually develop acutely inflamed thickened gallbladders. Acute hepatitis, usually secondary to viral infection, may mimic cholecystitis and/or cholangitis, with right upper quadrant abdominal pain, tenderness, vomiting, and fever. Children with hepatitis are frequently jaundiced. The results of liver function tests typically are markedly abnormal. Acute pancreatitis may mimic gallstone disease. In children, unlike adults, the most common causes of this condition are viral illness (some call this idiopathic pancreatitis) and blunt abdominal trauma. Often, one can elicit a history of recent viral illness (fever, myalgias, headache, vomiting) or, if the cause is traumatic, some sort of recent incident with blunt trauma, such as a motor vehicle crash or playground injury. Acute gastroenteritis (see discussion in Malrotation section) may mimic cholecystitis. Peptic ulcer disease or gastritis may present with more chronic symptoms and is difficult to distinguish from gallbladder disease. The pain tends to be more central (in the epigastrium) and more constant, and it may actually diminish with food intake (rather than worsen, as is typically the case with gallstone disease). Acute appendicitis also should be considered (see **Chapter 2**). Choledochal cyst disease also may resemble gallstone disease. It is a rare congenital anomaly of the biliary tree, with cystic dilation of the extrahepatic bile ducts.

Clinical Features

Most children with cholecystitis experience an acute onset of severe right upper quadrant or epigastric abdominal pain, typically 30 to 60 minutes after eating. The pain is usually sharp and may radiate around the right costal margin to the

back. It is typically associated with nausea, with or without vomiting, and may
be accompanied by fever. Murphy sign refers to right upper quadrant tenderness
to palpation when the patient is asked to take in a deep breath. The pain of
chronic cholecystitis is typically described as brief (lasting a few minutes),
self-resolving, chronic, and associated with eating fatty or greasy foods.

Cholecystitis can occur concomitantly with choledocholithiasis (passage of
gallstones into the common bile duct), cholangitis (bacterial infection of the
intrahepatic biliary tree because of bile duct obstruction), gallstone pancreatitis
(passage of a gallstone through the sphincter of Oddi), and even gallstone ileus
(adherence of an inflamed gallbladder to the intestinal tract, with bilioenteric
fistula formation). Thus, the stone can leave the gallbladder, travel distally
within the GI tract, and cause complete intestinal obstruction.

Evaluation

Blood tests include a complete blood cell count (with differential); liver function
tests, including alkaline phosphatase and total/direct bilirubin; and an assessment of pancreatic enzyme levels (amylase and lipase tests). Ultrasonography
is used to look for any stones, gallbladder wall thickening, or pericholecystic
fluid, as well as to reveal any tenderness when the gallbladder is compressed by
the transducer (radiographic Murphy sign). Children with cholecystitis also may
have choledocholithiasis if the laboratory evaluation reveals significant elevations of the bilirubin or pancreatic enzyme levels or if ultrasonography suggests
dilation of the biliary tree. Magnetic resonance cholangiopancreatography or
endoscopic retrograde cholangiopancreatography provides better visualization
of the biliary tree for evaluation and treatment of retained ductal stones.

Management

Children with acute cholecystitis are usually hospitalized for intravenous hydration and bowel rest. If fever or leukocytosis is present, intravenous antibiotics
should be administered. Preoperative management of patients with comorbid
sickle cell anemia may require the assistance of a pediatric hematologist.
Depending on the degree of inflammation, most children can be discharged
within 1 to 3 days after cholecystectomy.

Long-term Monitoring

Following cholecystectomy, most children have normal digestive patterns.
However, up to 10% of patients may experience diarrhea, which in rare
instances can be chronic. The exact mechanism is unclear. Recurrent gallstone
formation within the biliary tree is unusual, reportedly occurring in only 3%
to 5% of patients following surgery; some of these cases may actually involve

▼△▼△▼△▼△▼△▼△▼△▼　　▼△▼△▼△▼△▼△▼△▼△▼

individuals in whom gallstones were "left behind" in the stump of the cystic duct during cholecystectomy surgery.

OVARIAN TORSION

Overview/Definitions

Torsion is defined as twisting of the ovary on its vascular pedicle, which typically runs in the broad ligament beneath the fallopian tube. Torsion may occur prenatally if the female fetus develops an ovarian cyst from transplacental passage of maternal hormones. Most such ovaries infarct before birth and almost always require surgical removal. Although prenatal development of ovarian cysts is common, most such cysts are smaller than 4 to 5 cm in diameter and usually remain asymptomatic and resolve spontaneously.

Approximately half of ovarian torsions involve normal ovaries, while the other half are associated with ovarian pathology such as cysts and tumors (benign or malignant). Ovarian torsion can occur at any age, but it is far more common in adolescents than in younger children. The most common benign ovarian tumor causing torsion is the teratoma (also called an ovarian dermoid). Most pediatric ovarian torsions do not involve ovarian malignancies.

Differential Diagnosis

A ruptured ovarian cyst is most similar to an ovarian torsion. Girls with ruptured ovarian cysts have lower abdominal/pelvic pain that may be somewhat less sudden in onset (typically developing over several hours) and not as severe. Most ruptured cysts can be treated conservatively (with rest and pain medication), with gradual resolution of the pain. Acute appendicitis resembles torsion, but the pain with appendicitis typically develops much more gradually (over about 8–24 hours) and is usually associated with other gastrointestinal symptoms (nausea, vomiting) that are more pronounced. The first ovulation in an adolescent girl can result in symptoms quite similar to those in appendicitis, with localized pain, tenderness, and elevated white blood cell count. However, symptoms typically resolve on their own, within 1 to 2 days. Meckel diverticulitis may resemble ovarian torsion, but the pain typically develops much more gradually. Acute gastroenteritis also may mimic ovarian torsion but the gastrointestinal symptoms (nausea, vomiting, diarrhea) are typically much more pronounced and usually precede the pain.

Clinical Features

Most girls with ovarian torsion present with an acute onset of sharp, stabbing lower abdominal or pelvic pain. The pain is often constant but may subside somewhat if the child remains still. Nausea may be severe, with multiple episodes of vomiting. Fever is not usually present. Patients may have a history of milder symptoms.

Evaluation

Most cases of torsion can be diagnosed with ultrasonography, which may demonstrate an ovarian mass or a cyst or a swollen, enlarged ovary. Diminished color Doppler blood flow within the ovary may suggest torsion. However, the presence of Doppler flow does not exclude torsion.

Management

Suspected ovarian torsion usually requires urgent surgical intervention for attempted untwisting of the adnexa.

Long-term Monitoring

Patients undergo ultrasonography after 1 to 3 months for reevaluation, and then periodically for several years for assessment of ovarian size, shape, and blood flow. Even if serial ultrasound studies demonstrate that the detorsed ovary has atrophied, fertility rates in women with 1 ovary have not been shown to be significantly lower than rates in those with 2 ovaries (Evidence Level II-2).

RUPTURED OVARIAN CYSTS

Overview/Definitions

Ruptured ovarian cysts leak cyst fluid and/or blood into the peritoneal cavity, causing pain and other symptoms. Most cyst ruptures occur at the onset of puberty or during early adolescence when monthly ovarian hormonal cycles may be irregular or erratic. Most ruptured ovarian cysts do not require surgical intervention. Recurring ovarian cysts are common. Girls with polycystic ovary syndrome typically do not experience cyst rupture.

Causes

Most ruptured ovarian cysts are corpus luteum cysts, which are enlarged ovarian follicles that form during normal menstrual cycles. They are usually simple cysts, without multiple septae.

▼▲▼▲▼▲▼▲▼▲▼▲▼▲▼▲   ▲▼▲▼▲▼▲▼▲▼▲▼▲▼▲▼

Differential Diagnosis

The following conditions may mimic ovarian cyst rupture and have been discussed in detail earlier: ovarian torsion, acute appendicitis, ruptured Meckel diverticulitis, and acute gastroenteritis. Constipation may also resemble ovarian cyst rupture, but it is usually a chronic condition, with periodic exacerbations. The pain and tenderness of chronic constipation may be most severe in the right lower quadrant and are caused by stretching of the cecum. Plain abdominal radiographs may reveal significant stool retention and/or colonic dilation.

Evaluation

Most cysts can be detected by ultrasonography. Even small ovarian cysts (>2 cm diameter) can rupture in children, causing severe symptoms.

Management

If the diagnosis is clear, most ruptured ovarian cysts can be managed with oral analgesics (usually nonsteroidal anti-inflammatory drugs [NSAIDs]) and rest. Resolution of pain may take 3 to 5 days. Patients should be informed that ovarian cysts may develop again in the future. Occasionally, the patient's diagnostic workup is unclear, with the suspicion of possible acute appendicitis or ovarian torsion.

Long-term Monitoring

Because recurrence is common, patients and their families should be counseled about typical signs and symptoms. Mild pain attacks can usually be treated at home, with rest and NSAIDs. However, severe pain may indicate ovarian torsion or a different diagnosis (such as appendicitis), so severe pain should prompt consultation with a primary care provider.

SUGGESTED READING

Anders JF, Powell EC. Urgency of evaluation and outcome of acute ovarian torsion in pediatric patients. *Arch Pediatr Adolesc Med*. 2005;159(6):532–535

Garza JJ, Morash D, Dzakovic A, Mondschein JK, Jaksic T. Ad libitum feeding decreases hospital stay for neonates after pyloromyotomy. *J Pediatr Surg*. 2002;37(3):493–495

Graziano K, Islam S, Dasgupta R, et al. Asymptomatic malrotation: diagnosis and surgical management: an American Pediatric Surgical Association outcomes and evidence based practice committee systematic review. *J Pediatr Surg*. 2015;50(10):1783–1790

Guo JZ, Ma XY, Zhou QH. Results of air pressure enema reduction of intussusception: 6,396 cases in 13 years. *J Pediatr Surg*. 1986;21(12):1201–1203

Guthrie BD, Adler MD, Powell EC. Incidence and trends of pediatric ovarian torsion hospitalizations in the United States, 2000-2006. *Pediatrics*. 2010;125(3):532–538

Ito Y, Kusakawa I, Murata Y, et al. Japanese guidelines for the management of intussusception in children, 2011. *Pediatr Int*. 2012;54(6):948–958

Kaiser AD, Applegate KE, Ladd AP. Current success in the treatment of intussusception in children. *Surgery*. 2007;142(4):469–477

Kapfer SA, Rappold JF. Intestinal malrotation—not just the pediatric surgeon's problem. *J Am Coll Surg*. 2004;199(4):628–635

Kawahara H, Takama Y, Yoshida H, et al. Medical treatment of infantile hypertrophic pyloric stenosis: should we always slice the "olive"? *J Pediatr Surg*. 2005;40(12):1848–1851

Ko HS, Schenk JP, Tröger J, Rohrschneider WK. Current radiological management of intussusception in children. *Eur Radiol*. 2007;17(9):2411–2421

Kruatrachue A, Wongtapradit L, Nithipanya N, Ratanaprakarn W. Result of air enema reduction in 737 cases of intussusception. *J Med Assoc Thai*. 2011;94(Suppl 3):S22–S26

Mehall JR, Chandler JC, Mehall RL, Jackson RJ, Wagner CW, Smith SD. Management of typical and atypical intestinal malrotation. *J Pediatr Surg*. 2002;37(8):1169–1172

Mehta S, Lopez ME, Chumpitazi BP, Mazziotti MV, Brandt ML, Fishman DS. Clinical characteristics and risk factors for symptomatic pediatric gallbladder disease. *Pediatrics*. 2012;129(1):e82–e88

Michelotti B, Segura BJ, Sau I, Perez-Bertolez S, Prince JM, Kane TD. Surgical management of ovarian disease in infants, children, and adolescents: a 15-year review. *J Laparoendosc Adv Surg Tech A*. 2010;20(3):261–264

Naiditch JA, Rigsby C, Chin A. Delayed repeated enema and operative findings after unsuccessful primary enema for intussusception. *Eur J Pediatr Surg*. 2012;22(5):404–408

Oltmann SC, Fischer A, Barber R, Huang R, Hicks B, Garcia N. Pediatric ovarian malignancy presenting as ovarian torsion: incidence and relevance. *J Pediatr Surg*. 2010;45(1):135–139

Piper HG, Oltmann SC, Xu L, Adusumilli S, Fischer AC. Ovarian torsion: diagnosis of inclusion mandates earlier intervention. *J Pediatr Surg*. 2012;47(11):2071–2076

Poon TS, Zhang AL, Cartmill T, Cass DT. Changing patterns of diagnosis and treatment of infantile hypertrophic pyloric stenosis: a clinical audit of 303 patients. *J Pediatr Surg*. 1996; 31(12):1611–1615

Pryor HI 2nd, Lange PA, Bader A, Gilbert J, Newman K. Multiple magnetic foreign body ingestion: a surgical problem. *J Am Coll Surg*. 2007;205(1):182–186

Ruscher KA, Fisher JN, Hughes CD, et al. National trends in the surgical management of Meckel's diverticulum. *J Pediatr Surg*. 2011;46(5):893–896

Sharpe SJ, Rochette LM, Smith GA. Pediatric battery-related emergency department visits in the United States, 1990-2009. *Pediatrics*. 2012;129(6):1111–1117

Swaniker F, Soldes O, Hirschl RB. The utility of technetium 99m pertechnetate scintigraphy in the evaluation of patients with Meckel's diverticulum. *J Pediatr Surg*. 1999;34(5):760–765

Tessiatore P, Guanà R, Mussa A, et al. When to operate on ovarian cysts in children? *J Pediatr Endocrinol Metab.* 2012;25(5-6):427–433

Waltzman ML, Baskin M, Wypij D, Mooney D, Jones D, Fleisher G. A randomized clinical trial of the management of esophageal coins in children. *Pediatrics.* 2005;116(3):614–619

Abdominal Pain, Acute

John R. Stephens, MD, and Michael J. Steiner, MD, MPH

OVERVIEW

Abdominal pain is a common concern in the pediatric population in all clinical settings. Clinicians and research studies define acute abdominal pain as the onset of pain within 72 hours to 1 week of presentation. In this chapter, acute abdominal pain is differentiated from recurrent abdominal pain (repeated episodes of similar abdominal pain over a prolonged period) and chronic abdominal pain (pain that is usually or always present over a prolonged period) (see Chapter 3). Both recurrent and chronic abdominal pain can originate from diagnoses that overlap those for acute abdominal pain. However, once abdominal pain has recurred or persisted for a prolonged period, the most likely causes are different from the differential diagnoses associated with acute abdominal pain.

Most cases of acute abdominal pain arise from benign and self-limited conditions such as self-limiting abdominal pain or mild gastroenteritis (Evidence Level II-3). Some patients, however, have urgent and potentially life-threatening conditions.

Knowledge of the most common causes of abdominal pain in patients within certain age ranges can help focus preliminary diagnostic efforts (**Table 2-1**). A diagnostic challenge is that there are a wide variety of causes of abdominal pain within and outside the abdominal cavity. In many cases of diagnostic uncertainty, serial examinations are a reasonable and cost-effective approach.

CAUSES AND DIFFERENTIAL DIAGNOSIS

The differential diagnosis of abdominal pain is extremely broad, but it can be narrowed dramatically based on the patient's age, historical factors, and the preliminary physical examination findings (see **Table 2-1**). The most common diagnoses in emergency department settings are viral respiratory tract infections and group A streptococcal pharyngitis. Abdominal pain of unclear etiology,

Table 2-1. Differential Diagnosis of Acute Abdominal Pain Based on Age and Important Symptoms

	Infant	Toddler	School-aged Child	Adolescent
Specific symptoms	• Fever • Emesis: bilious or not • Stool pattern: frequency and quality of stool • Decreased feeding • Peritoneal symptoms or signs	• Fever • Emesis • Stool pattern: frequency and quality of stool • Decreased appetite • Dysuria • Peritoneal symptoms or signs	• Fever • Emesis • Stool pattern: frequency and quality of stool • Decreased appetite • Dysuria • Pain character: colicky or dull • Peritoneal symptoms or signs	• Fever • Emesis • Stool pattern: frequency and quality of stool • Decreased appetite • Dysuria • Menstrual history/ pregnancy status • Pain character: colicky or dull • Peritoneal symptoms or signs
Common nonsurgical abdominal diagnoses	• Urinary tract infection • Gastroenteritis • Colic • Infantile dyschezia • Milk protein allergy	• Nonspecific abdominal pain • Gastroenteritis • Constipation • Mesenteric adenitis	• Nonspecific abdominal pain • Gastroenteritis • Constipation • Mesenteric adenitis	• Nonspecific abdominal pain • Gastroenteritis • Constipation • Ruptured ovarian cyst • Pelvic inflammatory disease
Common surgical diagnoses	• Pyloric stenosis • Volvulus • Hernia • Trauma • Intussusception • Hirschsprung disease	• Intussusception • Appendicitis • Trauma • Swallowed foreign body	• Appendicitis • Trauma	• Appendicitis • Trauma • Ovarian/ testicular torsion • Ectopic pregnancy

	Infant	Toddler	School-aged Child	Adolescent
Non-abdominal or systemic causes	• Upper respiratory tract infection	• Upper respiratory tract infection • Pneumonia • Henoch-Schönlein purpura • Discitis	• Upper respiratory tract infection • Pharyngitis, group A strep-tococcal pharyngitis • Abdominal migraine • DKA • Pneumonia • Henoch-Schönlein purpura	• Upper respiratory tract infection • DKA • Pneumonia

Table 2-1. Differential Diagnosis of Acute Abdominal Pain Based on Age and Important Symptoms (*continued*)

Abbreviation: DKA, diabetic ketoacidosis.

other viral syndromes, and gastro-enteritis are frequent diagnoses. The most common diagnosis requiring surgical intervention is appendicitis (Evidence Level II-3).

CLINICAL FEATURES/SIGNS AND SYMPTOMS

Fever

Fever will increase or decrease the probability of a number of conditions. In infants, fever should raise the level of suspicion for urinary tract infection or gastroenteritis. In toddlers, fever raises the suspicion of urinary tract infection, along with respiratory infections, including lower lobe pneumonia, even in the absence of obvious respiratory symptoms. Diagnostic considerations for school-aged children with fever are similar, and group A streptococcal pharyngitis should also be considered. Fever in adolescent girls with abdominal pain raises the possibility of ascending sexually transmitted infections. In addition, fever can be associated with appendicitis and other conditions causing peritonitis. Absence of fever lowers the probability of appendicitis (Evidence Level III).

Vomiting

Emesis is an extremely important symptom. In infants, particular emphasis should be placed on the presence or absence of bilious emesis, as bile-stained vomitus suggests an obstructive process in the proximal small bowel and is highly suggestive of a morbid cause of pain. Bilious emesis in the neonate should prompt immediate evaluation with an upper gastrointestinal tract series and discussion with a pediatric surgeon. In older children, emesis is less likely to be caused by intestinal obstruction and most likely to be caused by acute gastroenteritis. Older children and adolescents occasionally develop bilious emesis after prolonged vomiting in the setting of a nonobstructive process. Classically, emesis will precede abdominal pain in gastroenteritis (Evidence Level III).

In contrast, with surgical causes of pain, such as appendicitis, pain tends to precede emesis, though this pattern is not reliably consistent (Evidence Level III).

Gastrointestinal

The stooling pattern is a key issue in a patient's medical history. In infants, straining with apparent discomfort during defecation, but resulting in soft stools and normal appearance at other times, is common. This pattern is seen with infantile dyschezia, a benign condition in infants learning to coordinate abdominal contractions with relaxation of rectal and pelvic floor musculature (Evidence Level III). Bloody stools in infants result most frequently from medical causes such as milk protein allergy. However, if the infant is distressed or appears ill, more serious causes, including intussusception, should be considered. Bloody stools in older children with abdominal pain should raise the clinician's level of suspicion for bacterial enteritis, although bowel necrosis from an urgent surgical diagnosis needs to be considered. Intussusception is observed most commonly in children during the second year after birth and typically causes episodic severe pain, often associated with crying and bending legs up to the abdomen. Diarrhea in all age ranges is associated with gastroenteritis but can accompany other conditions that cause abdominal pain. Lack of stool output can indicate constipation, but it also may reflect ileus or an anatomic intestinal obstruction and can be a subtle symptom of developing peritonitis (Evidence Level III).

Anorexia in older children is associated with appendicitis. In addition, it can be associated with bacterial disease such as streptococcal pharyngitis and pneumonia, as well as any severe systemic disease.

Pain

The characteristics of pain, including location, exacerbating factors, and intensity, can help make the diagnosis. Peritoneal symptoms tend to be subtle in children, especially infants. A child with peritonitis is often less active; children who writhe during the examination are less likely to have peritonitis. A history of increased pain with movement, such as driving in a car over rough roads, is important, and eliciting this information may require clinicians to ask parents directly (Evidence Level III).

Older children can have the same patterns as those observed in infants and toddlers, but pain preceding emesis is somewhat more suggestive of a condition that may need surgical treatment.

EVALUATION

The physical examination should begin with the child in a comfortable position away from the examiner. The examiner should note the child's overall appearance and if the patient is walking or moving normally, moving frequently, or lying still. The clinician should focus on the abdomen toward the end of the examination but before other, uncomfortable, examination elements. Focusing on the anatomic structures located near the abdomen, including the lung bases superior to the abdomen and the genitalia and hips inferior to the abdomen, is particularly important. The abdominal examination may start with auscultation of bowel sounds followed by palpation of the abdomen. There are varying attitudes among clinicians about how frequently a rectal examination is needed to help establish a diagnosis in a child with abdominal pain. In cases with no definitive diagnosis suggested by symptoms or initial evaluation, a rectal examination can provide additional diagnostic information. Similarly, a gynecologic examination is rarely needed, but if vaginal discharge or lower abdominal pain and fever in an adolescent are present, a pelvic examination can be critical. Appendicitis is the most common diagnosis of acute abdominal pain that requires surgery for patients of all ages except infants (Evidence Level II-3). In some case series in emergency departments, up to 10% of children with abdominal pain have been reported to have appendicitis. However, in a case series composed of more than 1,000 children who attended an urgent care setting or emergency department at a large children's hospital, slightly less than 1% of those older than 2 years with a chief concern of abdominal pain had appendicitis (Evidence Level II-3). History and physical examination findings are most helpful when grouped in a clinical scoring system. The most commonly studied system is the Alvarado score (**Table 2-2**), which assigns points for specific signs, symptoms, and laboratory values.

In cases of diagnostic uncertainty, laboratory tests for complete blood cell count, erythrocyte sedimentation rate, C-reactive protein concentration, and urinalysis are usually ordered. Other laboratory tests evaluating for liver or pancreatic inflammation, genitourinary tract infections, or pregnancy should be used in appropriate clinical scenarios. Radiologic imaging should focus

▼▲▼▲▼▲▼▲▼▲▼▲▼▲▼▲▼▲ ▼▲▼▲▼▲▼▲▼▲▼▲▼▲▼▲▼

Table 2-2. Alvarado Score for Appendicitis (Note the MANTRELS Mnemonic)

	Feature	Value
Symptoms	Migration Anorexia Nausea/vomiting	1 1 1
Signs	Tenderness in right lower quadrant Rebound pain Elevated temperature	2 1 1
Laboratory values	Leukocytosis Shift of white blood cell count to the left	2 1
Total score[a]		**10**

[a] Scores >7 points have a positive likelihood ratio that approximates 4.0 (CI, 3.2 to 4.9) and scores ≤4 reflect a dramatically decreased likelihood of appendicitis, with a likelihood ratio of 0.05 (CI, 0.0 to 0.85).

Reprinted with permission from Alvarado A. A practical score for the early diagnosis of acute appendicitis. *Ann Emerg Med.* 1986;15(5):557–564.

on diagnosing or excluding specific conditions, rather than serve as a broad diagnostic tool in the undifferentiated patient (Evidence Level III).

Infant

Laboratory Tests

To exclude a urinary tract infection, the physician should order a catheterized urinalysis for the febrile infant. Stool antigen testing for rotavirus can be diagnostic in the setting of acute diarrheal illness, though management of the disease is not altered by this result (Evidence Level III).

Radiologic Imaging

Plain abdominal radiographs, particularly those with a supine and an upright or a lateral view, are helpful in the evaluation of suspected obstructive processes or if signs of peritonitis are present to exclude a perforated viscus. Radiographs can suggest an intussusception but generally are not diagnostic. Ultrasonography performed in experienced centers can diagnose intussusception; however, an air or a contrast (preferably water soluble) enema will be both diagnostic and therapeutic. The clinician should order an upper gastrointestinal tract contrast study when malrotation with volvulus or another proximal intestinal obstruction is suspected, usually in the presence of bilious emesis. Contrast enema is the test of choice in the acute setting when Hirschsprung disease is suspected because it is often the easiest to obtain. Guidelines suggest that anorectal manometry is a preferred diagnostic method for Hirschsprung disease in nonacute settings, but it is not immediately available in most centers. Abnormal contrast enema findings reveal a transition point from a normal-sized rectum to a dilated sigmoid colon. No rectal manipulation should be done in the 24 hours preceding this test to avoid temporarily dilating the transition point (Evidence Level III). Rectal biopsy can also be performed as a primary diagnostic test for children with symptoms that are highly suggestive of Hirschsprung disease.

One to 5 Years of Age

Laboratory Tests

Urinalysis should be considered for the febrile patient. Group A streptococcal pharyngitis testing also should be considered. Physicians should consider rotavirus testing in patients with diarrheal illness. Blood tests can be a useful adjunct in diagnosing acute appendicitis. A peripheral white blood cell (WBC) count of less than 10,000/μL lowers the posttest odds of appendicitis by 80% (likelihood ratio of 0.22), whereas a WBC count of greater than 10,000/μL doubles the posttest odds (likelihood ratio of 2.0) (Evidence Level II-2).

Radiologic Imaging

Plain radiographs of the abdomen may aid in evaluating the patient for constipation or when the history or physical examination findings suggest obstruction or peritonitis. The physician should consider obtaining a plain radiograph of the chest for a febrile patient, with or without respiratory symptoms, to exclude lower lobe pneumonia if no other cause of fever is apparent. Experienced centers may perform ultrasonography to look for intussusception (Evidence Level II-2). We should point out that the accuracy of ultrasonography in diagnosing appendicitis is highly operator dependent. An upper gastrointestinal tract contrast study should be performed when malrotation with volvulus or another proximal intestinal obstruction is suspected. Cases of intussusception can be diagnosed and treated with an air or a contrast enema. Computed tomography can be used to diagnose acute appendicitis reliably, but it is time-consuming and expensive and exposes the patient to significant radiation (Evidence Level III).

School-aged Child

Considerations are similar to those for preschool-aged children, except that volvulus and intussusception are much less common, and patients generally can provide a more detailed history and are more tolerant of a physical examination.

Adolescent

Additional considerations include pregnancy and its complications, sexually transmitted infections, menstrual- and ovulation-related pain, and gonadal torsion.

Laboratory Tests

Urinalysis should be considered for patients with symptoms of urinary frequency, dysuria, or hematuria. A urine pregnancy test should be considered for girls who are post-menarche. Urine also can be tested for sexually transmitted infections, and purulent urethral or vaginal discharges can be tested for gonorrheal and chlamydial disease (Evidence Level III).

Radiologic Imaging

Ultrasonography with views of vascular structures when appropriate is often critical to diagnose genitourinary tract conditions, including ovarian torsion, ectopic pregnancy, and testicular torsion.

MANAGEMENT

Treatment depends on the underlying diagnosis. A firm diagnosis may not be possible even after a careful history, physical examination, and directed ancillary testing. In such cases, nonspecific abdominal pain is likely the diagnosis, and close follow-up or serial abdominal examinations may be the best course.

Several indications call for a pediatric surgical consultation, including signs or symptoms of peritonitis; intestinal obstruction, especially bilious or feculent emesis; incarcerated inguinal hernia; and any suggestion of a cause necessitating surgical treatment on radiologic imaging, such as free air in the peritoneum (Evidence Level III).

A frequent reason for surgical consultation is suspected appendicitis. When a presumptive diagnosis of appendicitis is made, broad-spectrum antibiotics (eg, piperacillin/tazobactam) should be prescribed pending an appendectomy (Evidence Level III).

Withholding pain medications in children with severe acute abdominal pain for fear of "masking" is not supported by medical evidence, and, in fact, adequate pain control may enhance diagnostic accuracy by allowing a more thorough physical examination (Evidence Level I). Acetaminophen is a reasonable choice in patients who can take oral medications and have mild-to-moderate pain, while weight-based intravenous morphine or fentanyl (not to exceed an adult dose) is safe and effective for children who are unable to tolerate oral dosing or for those who have more severe pain.

SUGGESTED READING

Bundy DG, Byerley JS, Liles EA, Perrin EM, Katznelson J, Rice HE. Does this child have appendicitis? *JAMA*. 2007;298(4):438–451

Green R, Bulloch B, Kabani A, Hancock BJ, Tenenbein M. Early analgesia for children with acute abdominal pain. *Pediatrics*. 2005;116(4):978–983

Kosloske A, Love CL, Rohrer JE, Goldthorn JF, Lacey SR. The diagnosis of appendicitis in children: outcomes of a strategy based on pediatric surgical evaluation. Pediatrics. 2004;113(1):29–34

Ross A, LeLeiko NS. Acute abdominal pain. *Pediatr Rev*. 2010;31(4):135–144

Saito JM. Beyond appendicitis: evaluation and surgical treatment of pediatric acute abdominal pain. *Curr Opin Pediatr*. 2012;24(3):357–364

Scholer SJ, Pituch K, Orr DP, Dittus RS. Clinical outcomes of children with acute abdominal pain. *Pediatrics*. 1996;98(4):680–685

Abdominal Pain, Functional

Nader N. Youssef, MD

OVERVIEW

The Rome criteria for the diagnosis of functional abdominal pain (FAP)-related disorders have been updated. Functional abdominal pain usually refers to pain alone, while irritable bowel syndrome (IBS) usually refers to abdominal pain with disordered defecation (ie, constipation, diarrhea). Abdominal pain with bloating is often referred to as *nonulcer dyspepsia*. Despite the differences in terminology, FAP and irritable bowel syndrome (IBS) remain closely related disorders.

THE PEDIATRIC ROME IV CRITERIA: UPDATE

In 2016, the symptom-based criteria used to diagnose functional gastrointestinal disorders (FGIDs), known as the Rome criteria, were revised and published as the Rome IV criteria. For children and adolescents, the 3 categories of FGIDs are functional nausea and vomiting disorders, functional abdominal pain disorders, and functional defecation disorders. The updated criteria state that the diagnosis of these disorders can be made only if "after appropriate medical evaluation, the symptoms cannot be attributed to another medical condition." Previously, a diagnosis could be made only if there was "no evidence of an inflammatory, anatomic, metabolic, or neoplastic process that explains the subject's symptoms," often requiring more intensive evaluation such as endoscopy or advanced imaging studies. This change should reduce the testing needed for a FGID diagnosis.

Rome IV Criteria for Diagnosis: Functional Abdominal Pain– Not Otherwise Specified

Symptoms that support the FAP–not otherwise specified diagnosis must be present for at least 6 months, occur at least 4 times per month, and include all of the following: (1) episodic or continuous abdominal pain that does not occur solely during physiologic events such as eating or menses, (2) insufficient criteria for IBS, functional dyspepsia (early satiety and postprandial fullness are the hallmarks), or abdominal migraine (episodic severe pain lasting at least 1 hour and associated with headache, photophobia, pallor, and interference with activities including a need to rest), and (3) after appropriate evaluation, the abdominal pain cannot be fully explained by another medical condition.

Rome IV Criteria for Diagnosis: Irritable Bowel Syndrome

A diagnosis of IBS is supported by symptoms that are present for at least 2 months, including abdominal pain at least 4 days per month associated with 1 or more of the following: defecation, a change in the frequency of stool, and a change in the form or appearance of stool. In children with constipation, the pain persists despite treatment. The revised criteria retain language stating that after an appropriate evaluation, a diagnosis of IBS can be made only if the symptoms cannot be fully explained by another medical condition. This criterion often can be met with a limited evaluation, such as screening blood work and stool studies.

CAUSES AND DIFFERENTIAL DIAGNOSIS

The etiology of FAP is largely unknown. Pathophysiologic evidence suggests several potential mechanisms for abdominal pain in functional bowel disorders: altered intestinal motility, altered intestinal sensory thresholds to distention or tissue damage, genetic predisposition, and psychosocial factors such as vulnerability and coping style. Other factors that have been shown to contribute to persistent FAP include family stress, early life events (ie, abuse), and environmental factors (recurrent infection or use of antibiotics).

All these factors may be related to the key area of brain-gut axis research. It is now well recognized that a bidirectional signaling exists between the gut and brain. When alternations occur in these pathways, there is a propensity for gastrointestinal dysfunction. Recent studies using functional magnetic resonance imaging (fMRI) of the brain have demonstrated structural and functional differences between children with IBS and healthy controls.

CLINICAL AND LABORATORY EVALUATION

One of the more novel features of the updated Rome IV criteria is the development of the Multi-Dimensional Clinical Profile (MDCP) and Interactive Clinical Decision Toolkit, which are software programs that incorporate the diagnostic algorithms and the MDCP. The MDCP is a learning module that helps clinicians

▼△▼△▼△▼△▼△▼△▼△▼△▼△ ▼△▼△▼△▼△▼△▼△▼△▼△▼

better understand the FGIDs. A key feature of the MDCP is that it forces the clinician to answer questions about illness severity, psychological comorbidity, and potential underlying pathophysiology that may be occurring at the time of evaluation. Use of these tools may lead to more directed therapies.

Box 3-1 lists a limited set of laboratory investigations to aid in screening for intestinal inflammation and malabsorption. A comprehensive metabolic panel may help identify patients with conditions such as liver disorders. Screening for celiac disease includes total IgA level and tissue transglutaminase and anti-endomysial antibodies. An abdominal radiograph can reveal occult constipation as a cause of recurrent abdominal pain. A hydrogen breath test will evaluate for lactase deficiency as a cause of symptoms. Physicians should include stool testing for parasites (eg, *Giardia, Cyclospora cayetanensis,* and *Isospora*) and infections (eg, *Clostridium difficile, Salmonella, Shigella, Campylobacter jejuni*) in the workup. Screening for systemic inflammation includes a determination of the sedimentation rate or C-reactive protein concentration; in addition, stool testing for fecal calprotectin identifies inflammation within the intestine. This test helps to differentiate IBS from inflammatory conditions such as Crohn disease (Evidence Level II-1). However, a history consistent with diarrhea accompanied by weight loss, blood in the stools, recurrent fevers, mouth sores, or suspected nutritional deficiency should prompt an investigation—including endoscopy—for intestinal disease to rule out an

Box 3-1. Limited Evaluation for Functional Abdominal Pain

- Abdominal radiograph (only if constipation is suspected and to assess for impaction)
- Total IgA level and anti-endomysial antibodies
- C-reactive protein concentration
- Complete blood cell count
- Comprehensive metabolic panel
- Erythrocyte sedimentation rate
- Fecal calprotectin level
- Stool testing for infection, including ova, parasites, *Helicobacter pylori,* and *Clostridium difficile*
- Tissue transglutaminase level

infection or a mucosal pathology, such as inflammatory bowel disease, Crohn disease, or ulcerative colitis.

MANAGEMENT

Conventional Approach

Current treatment for children with FAP is to reassure the child and family that no serious progressive disease is present, that they eventually will outgrow the symptoms, and that the child must learn coping techniques. Pharmaceutical treatments are commonly used to manage symptoms of FAP in childhood despite the lack of data supporting their efficacy. These approaches include use of fiber, antacids, and antispasmodics. Probiotics with certain beneficial strains such as *Lactobacillus* GG, VSL#3, and *Bifidobacterium* may be considered for a short trial period. Physicians can consider a low-FODMAPs (fermentable oligosaccharides, disaccharides, monosaccharides, and polyols) diet when the symptoms of pain are associated with bloating, and a diet history revealing high intake of fermentable carbohydrates can be established (Evidence Level II-2).

Innovative Approaches

In adults, low-dose antidepressants have been useful in the management of irritable bowel disease. The role of amitriptyline as a monotherapy for FAP in children continues be unclear, and it is currently reserved for those who may have overlapping anxiety or depression associated with significant disabling pain. In such cases, amitriptyline is used along with psychological intervention to emphasize more meaningful coping as part of the child's recovery (Evidence Level I).

Integrative Medicine Intervention

Studies have shown that many children (36%) visiting a gastroenterologist for the first time are already following a complementary and alternative medicine (CAM) regimen. Seventy-three percent of the parents of these children attributed symptomatic improvements to CAM. Interventions included over-the-counter products, spiritual practices, visits to alternative practitioners, and dietary modifications (Evidence Level II-3). Over-the-counter products and dietary modifications ranked moderate on patient satisfaction scales, while spiritual practices and alternative practitioner visits ranked highest. Other CAM practices, such as oral supplementation, acupuncture, aromatherapy, and osteopathic manipulation, are popular among adults with FAP.

▼▲▼▲▼▲▼▲▼▲▼▲▼▲▼▲▼   ▲▼▲▼▲▼▲▼▲▼▲▼▲▼▲▼

Guided Imagery or Hypnotherapy

Conventional treatment for FAP is largely unsatisfactory. Increasing evidence shows that mind/body approaches are quite useful in treating FAP in children. Guided imagery, self-hypnosis, or strategies aimed at improving coping skills have become first-line therapies for most pediatric gastroenterologists who are asked to evaluate children with FAP. These therapies are applicable to all children with FAP regardless of severity (Evidence Level II-1). Studies in children and adolescents have reported significantly lower abdominal pain levels in those who visited individual therapists, participated in group classes, or used self-guided CDs. Positive effects have been reported to persist for up to 5 years.

Role of Family and Parental Intervention

Several investigators have reported reduced abdominal pain, improved quality of life, and lower school absenteeism when both the child and family members are treated concurrently. Often, a formal program that focuses on identifying parental worries and modifying behavior can be helpful. Programs should address the additional comorbidities that often exist, such as anxiety and/or depression, and secondary issues, such as learned impaired eating (ie, refusal to eat because of pain, or fear of vomiting/diarrhea). Education about brain-gut connections are key issues for parents and other family members. Strategies to reduce the frequency of parental inquiries about abdominal pain have shown promise in leading to overall behavioral change in children with FAP.

Role of Diet

Dietary intake is another possible cause of symptoms related to FAP. In fact, at least two-thirds of adults with IBS, as well as two-thirds of children with functional gastrointestinal disorders, perceive their symptoms to be food related, making dietary management an important tool in the treatment of IBS (Evidence Level II-2). In the past few years, there has been increasing interest in a low FODMAPs diet, which decreases the intake of many fermentable carbohydrates. The FODMAPs foods include such items as pears, apples, wheat, onion, legumes, stone fruits, and artificial sweeteners. Some evidence suggests a modest benefit from a FODMAPs-restricted diet in children with IBS; this benefit may be related to reduced distention from gas-producing gut bacteria and an improved gut flora. While this diet may be effective as a treatment approach for some patients, it can be difficult to adhere to and requires significant family support.

▼△▼△▼△▼△▼△▼△▼△▼△▼   ▼△▼△▼△▼△▼△▼△▼△▼△▼

LONG-TERM CONSIDERATIONS

Evidence shows that FAP is rarely a self-limiting condition; after 5 years, one-third of children continue to experience symptoms (**Figure 3-1**). Children with FAP can have significant school absence, family disruption, and social withdrawal, with tendencies toward anxiety and depression. Such morbidity can result in an impaired quality of life. In addition, children with FAP continue to utilize health care services at an increased rate in young adulthood.

Children with FAP may experience symptoms for more than 1 year before adequate relief is achieved. Patients with FGIDs also may have sleep difficulties, headaches, dizziness, and fatigue.

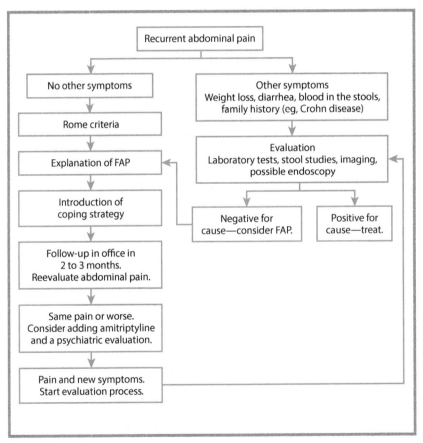

Figure 3-1. Functional Abdominal Pain Algorithm

Abbreviation: FAP, functional abdominal pain.

SUGGESTED READING

Chitkara DK, Talley NJ, Weaver AL, et al. Incidence of presentation of common functional gastro-intestinal disorders in children from birth to 5 years: a cohort study. *Clin Gastroenterol Hepatol.* 2007;5(2):186–191

Di Lorenzo C, Youssef NN, Sigurdsson L, Scharff L, Griffiths J, Wald A. Visceral hyperalgesia in children with functional abdominal pain. *J Pediatr.* 2001;139(6):838–843

Hyams JS, Burke G, Davis PM, Rzepski B, Andrulonis PA. Abdominal pain and irritable bowel syndrome in adolescents: a community-based study. *J Pediatr.* 1996;129(2):220–226

Hyams JS, Di Lorenzo C, Saps M, Shulman RJ, Staiano A, van Tilburg M. Functional disorders: children and adolescents. *Gastroenterology.* 2016;150(6):1456–1468.e2

Koppen IJ, Nurko S, Saps M, Di Lorenzo C, Benninga MA. The pediatric Rome IV criteria: what's new? *Expert Rev Gastroenterol Hepatol.* 2017;11(3):193–201

Rutten JM, Korternik JJ, Venmans LM, Benninga MA, Tabbers MM. Nonpharmacologic treatment of functional abdominal pain disorders: a systematic review. *Pediatrics.* 2015;135(3):522–535

Saps M, Youssef N, Miranda A, et al. Multicenter, randomized, placebo-controlled trial of amitripty-line in children with functional gastrointestinal disorders. *Gastroenterology.* 2009;137(4):1261–1269

Turco R, Salvatore S, Miele E, Romano C, Marseglia GL, Staiano A . Does a low FODMAPs diet reduce symptoms of functional abdominal pain disorders? A systematic review in adult and paediat-ric population, on behalf of Italian Society of Pediatrics. *Ital J Pediatr.* 2018;44(1):53

Varni JW, Lane MM, Burwinkle TM, et al. Health-related quality of life in pediatric patients with irritable bowel syndrome: a comparative analysis. *J Dev Behav Pediatr.* 2006;27(6):451–458

Vlieger AM, Menko-Frankenhuis C, Wolfkamp SC, Tromp E, Benninga M. Hypnotherapy for children with functional abdominal pain or irritable bowel syndrome: a randomized controlled trial. *Gastroenterology.* 2007;133(5):1430–1436

Youssef NN, Murphy TG, Langseder AL, Rosh JR. Quality of life for children with functional abdominal pain: a comparison study of patients' and parents' perceptions. *Pediatrics.* 2006;117(1):54–59

Youssef NN, Rosh JR, Loughran M, et al. Treatment of functional abdominal pain in childhood with cognitive behavioral strategies. *J Pediatr Gastroenterol Nutr.* 2004;39(2):192–196

Celiac Disease

Karl Horvath, MD, PhD

OVERVIEW

Celiac disease (CD) is an autoimmune enteropathy that develops in genetically susceptible individuals and is the result of an immune reaction to gluten, found in wheat, barley, rye, and related grains. Treatment for CD is elimination of gluten from the diet, which typically results in full mucosal recovery in children. Compliance with the diet eliminates the morbidity and mortality associated with untreated CD. Children younger than 2 years can develop classical malabsorptive symptoms within months of being on a gluten containing diet.

CAUSES AND DIFFERENTIAL DIAGNOSIS

Celiac disease leads to intestinal villus atrophy and a subsequent decrease in the intestinal absorptive surface and malabsorption of nutrients. The differential diagnosis includes other diseases that result in malabsorption (**Table 4-1**).

CLINICAL FEATURES/SIGNS AND SYMPTOMS

The classic clinical symptoms of CD include weight loss, anemia, diarrhea, bloating, gaseousness, muscle weakness, short stature, and appetite changes (**Box 4-1**). One study reported that only 1 in 7 children diagnosed with CD had these classic symptoms (Evidence Level II-2). The term *celiac iceberg* was introduced based on that study, which determined that the classic cases represented only the tip of the iceberg. Therefore, serologic screening is necessary in individuals who do not have classic symptoms, but are suspected of having CD. **Box 4-2** shows diseases and conditions that should prompt further testing for CD.

In 2011, a multidisciplinary task force of physicians classified patients into several groups based on their symptoms, histology, CD serology, and genetic test results (**Table 4-2**).

▼▲▼▲▼▲▼▲▼▲▼▲▼▲▼▲▼ ▼▲▼▲▼▲▼▲▼▲▼▲▼▲▼▲▼

Table 4-1. Differential Diagnosis of Celiac Disease

Pathomechanism	Diseases
Digestive enzyme deficiency without mucosal damage	Lactose malabsorption Sucrase-isomaltase deficiency Other disaccharidase deficiencies Pancreatic insufficiencies: cystic fibrosis, chronic pancreatitis; isolated enzyme deficiencies (lipase, amylase)
Digestive enzyme inactivation	Zollinger-Ellison syndrome
Transport defects	Fructose malabsorption Abetalipoproteinemia
Mucosal damage	Autoimmune enteropathy Crohn disease NSAID enteropathy Radiation enteritis
Infectious causes	*Giardia* infestation Tropical sprue Cryptosporiasis (HIV)
Anatomical/motility problems	Pseudo-obstruction Small bowel microbial overgrowth
Allergy/immunology	Cow's milk protein intolerance Eosinophilic gastroenteritis Autoimmune enteropathy

Abbreviation: NSAID, nonsteroidal anti-inflammatory drug.

Classic cases more likely manifest in children between the ages of 9 and 24 months if gluten has been introduced into the diet. In children older than 2 years, classic symptoms are reported less frequently, probably because their intestinal adaptation is better. The average age at diagnosis has shifted well above the toddler years, and many children with newly diagnosed CD have no classic symptoms.

About 8% to 15% of children with idiopathic short stature have CD without any digestive symptoms (see **Box 4-1**).

First- and second-degree relatives of patients with CD may have a subclinical form of the disease. The wide spectrum of clinical manifestations and the strong association with other autoimmune (eg, diabetes) and genetic (eg, Down syndrome) diseases are well known (**Box 4-3**).

Box 4-1. Typical Signs and Symptoms of Celiac Disease

- Weight loss
- Failure to thrive
- Chronic or intermittent diarrhea
- Chronic abdominal pain, cramping
- Abdominal distension
- Gaseousness/bloating

Box 4-2. Diseases and Conditions Prompting Testing for Celiac Disease

- First-degree relatives of children with CD
- Type 1 diabetes mellitus
- Down syndrome
- Autoimmune thyroid disease
- Turner syndrome
- Williams syndrome
- Selective IgA deficiency
- Autoimmune liver disease

EVALUATION

It is important to emphasize that no CD exists if gluten has never been added to the diet. If serologic test results suggest CD, referral to a pediatric gastroenterologist is necessary to confirm the diagnosis with an intestinal biopsy based on the North American expert guidelines. A repeated intestinal biopsy to confirm the histologic recovery on a gluten-free diet (GFD) is not necessary (Evidence Level III).

Table 4-2. Oslo Definitions of Celiac Disease

Oslo Definitions	Symptoms	HLA DQ2 and/or HLA DQ8	Histology	Serology
Classic CD	Diarrhea, bloating, weight loss, nutritional deficiencies, failure to thrive, muscle wasting, signs of emotional distress, and lethargy	Present	Abnormal	Abnormal
Nonclassic CD	No signs or symptoms of malabsorption but various nonclassic manifestations (see **Box 4-3**)	Present	Abnormal	Abnormal
Subclinical CD	No signs or symptoms sufficient to trigger CD testing in routine practice but patient is at-risk for CD	Present	Abnormal	Abnormal
Potential CD	No signs or symptoms; normal small intestinal mucosa but positive CD serology	Present	Normal	Abnormal
Refractory CD	Persistent or recurrent malabsorptive symptoms and villus atrophy despite a strict gluten-free diet (GFD) for more than 12 months	Present	Remains abnormal despite GFD	Abnormal but becomes normal on GFD

Abbreviation: CD, celiac disease.

Derived from Ludvigsson JF, Leffler DA, Bai JC, et al. The Oslo definitions for coeliac disease and related terms. *Gut.* 2013;62(1):43–52.

Serology Tests

The presence of celiac-specific antibodies is crucial not only for the diagnosis, but also because they provide baseline laboratory results that enable the physician to assess the child's response to the GFD. IgA and IgG antibody-based tests are available, but the IgA antibody tests have higher sensitivity and specificity.

▼▲▼▲▼▲▼▲▼▲▼▲▼▲▼ ▲▼▲▼▲▼▲▼▲▼▲▼▲▼▲▼

Box 4-3. Nonclassic Presentations of Celiac Disease

- Dermatitis herpetiformis
- Short stature
- Delayed puberty
- Refractory iron deficiency anemia
- Recurrent aphthous stomatitis
- Dental enamel hypoplasia
- Osteoporosis/osteopenia
- Hypertransaminasemia
- Partial focal temporal epilepsy
- Alopecia
- Ataxia
- Polyneuropathy
- Irritable bowel syndrome
- Iron deficiency anemia
- Constipation

Antigliadin and Deamidated Antigliadin Antibodies

The deamidated gliadin peptide (DGP) tests have better sensitivity and specificity than the traditional antigliadin tests but they lag the tissue transglutaminase (tTG) IgA and endomysium antibody (EmA) IgA tests (Evidence Level III).

Endomysium Antibody Test

The combination of the antigliadin and EmA tests has a 99.6% positive predictive value for the presence of flat mucosa. In children younger than 2 years, the EmA IgA can be negative; therefore, an intestinal biopsy is necessary if symptoms and an elevated antigliadin or DGP antibody are present.

Tissue Transglutaminase Antibody Tests

The sensitivity and specificity of the IgA tTG test are comparable to those of the IgA EmA test (Evidence Level II-3). The IgA tTG test is the recommended first screening test for CD (Evidence Level III.) Selective IgA-deficient patients with IgG type EmA or tTG IgG elevations need to undergo a biopsy of the small

▼▲▼▲▼▲▼▲▼▲▼▲▼▲▼   ▲▼▲▼▲▼▲▼▲▼▲▼▲▼

intestine to rule out CD. The tTG IgA test can be falsely positive in children with autoimmune disorders (eg, children with diabetes mellitus).

Genetic (HLA DQ2/DQ8) Tests

HLA-DQ2 and HLA-DQ8 typing is useful to exclude CD as it has a high negative predictive value. HLA testing is recommended in patients in whom the diagnosis of CD is uncertain. It has a role in screening asymptomatic but at-risk individuals, such as first-degree relatives, children with type 1 diabetes, and those with Down syndrome, Turner syndrome, and Williams syndrome. The absence of the HLA DQ2/DQ8 haplotypes renders CD highly unlikely; therefore, HLA testing is cost-effective in these patients because most can be excluded from further periodic serology studies (Evidence Level III).

Intestinal Biopsy

Intestinal biopsy is considered the gold standard in the diagnosis of CD (Evidence Level III). The individual histologic changes are not specific for CD and may be found in other enteropathies; however, in combination with serologic test findings, they confirm the diagnosis.

According to the Modified Marsh Classification scale, the degree of histologic changes in CD is classified as follows:
- Type 1: infiltrative lesion (normal height of villi but increased intraepithelial lymphocytes)
- Type 2: hyperplastic lesion (type 1 plus elongated, hyperplastic crypts)
- Type 3: destructive lesion (elongated crypts plus progressively worse villus atrophy) (3a, mild atrophy; 3b, marked atrophy; and 3c, total flattening of the villi).

There is good evidence that the mucosal changes in CD may be patchy in nature and vary in severity; therefore, multiple endoscopic biopsy specimens (4 to 6) should be obtained from the duodenal bulb and distal segments of the duodenum (Evidence Level III). All of the histologic abnormalities should completely resolve after the elimination of gluten from the diet. In most cases, it is unnecessary to repeat the small-bowel biopsies in children on a GFD to confirm the intestinal mucosal recovery (Evidence Level III). However, if there are persistent symptoms or poor growth and a dietary transgression is excluded, then a repeat endoscopy is indicated.

▼▲▼▲▼▲▼▲▼▲▼▲▼▲▼ ▼▲▼▲▼▲▼▲▼▲▼▲▼▲▼

MANAGEMENT

Six areas require monitoring, as discussed herein.

Gluten-Free Diet

It is important not to initiate a GFD before a pediatric gastroenterologist confirms the diagnosis, as the mucosal damage will improve, making the histologic diagnosis more difficult. After the diagnosis is confirmed by means of an intestinal biopsy, the child and his or her entire family should receive professional dietary counseling for a GFD. Within 12 months after starting the GFD, the antibody titers should decline below the cutoff values.

Evidence shows that diagnosed but untreated CD is associated with a significant increase in morbidity and mortality in adults (Evidence Level II-2). Prolonged adherence to a GFD reduces the risks of morbidity and mortality to those found in the general population (Evidence Level II-3).

The current treatment for CD is a life-long GFD, with elimination of wheat, rye, barley, and related grains. A diet guideline developed by an expert panel is available (www.gastrokids.org). Multiple studies have found that pure, noncontaminated oat flour can be consumed by most patients with CD (Evidence Level II-3).

One of the major difficulties in following the GFD is that the 3 main grains have been modified and are produced under different names (eg, triticale, a combination of wheat and rye), kamut, and spelt (sometimes called *faro*). Other forms of wheat are semolina (durum wheat), einkorn, bulgur, and couscous. Malt is also toxic because it is a partial hydrolysate of barley prolamins. **Box 4-4** lists the gluten-containing and gluten-free grains.

According to the Codex Alimentarius, gluten-free foods are foods or ingredients in which the measured gluten level is less than 20 ppm. In an Italian study of adults with CD, some patients tolerated 34 to 36 mg of gluten per day, while others who consumed about 10 mg of gluten per day developed mucosal abnormalities. Therefore, a daily gluten intake of less than 10 mg is unlikely to cause histologic changes.

The follow-up clinic visits involve the assessment of clinical symptoms, discussion of the results of repeated celiac serology tests, treatment of nutritional deficiencies, checking growth parameters, and nutritional counseling. Reports indicate that more than one-half of children with CD did not develop immunity to hepatitis B despite receiving vaccination at birth. Therefore, checking the hepatitis B surface antibody titer in newly diagnosed cases is advisable (Evidence Level II-3).

Box 4-4. Grains That Contain Gluten and Those That Are Allowed in the Gluten-Free Diet

Well-known grains containing gluten	Other grains that contain gluten	Gluten-free grains
• Wheat	• Bulgur	• Amaranth
• Wheat bran	• Couscous	• Arrowroot
• Wheat starch	• Durum	• Buckwheat
• Wheat germ	• Emmer	• Corn
• Barley	• Einkorn	• Flax
• Barley malt extract	• Faro	• Millet
• Rye	• Filler	• Montina
	• Kamut	• Oat
	• Semolina	• Quinoa
	• Spelt	• Rice
	• Triticale	• Sorghum
		• Tapioca
		• Teff

Lactose Malabsorption

Approximately 80% to 90% of children with Marsh type 3 lesions have abnormally low lactase activity, which is secondary to the mucosal damage and may require a few weeks to resolve. Consequently, newly diagnosed children should follow a low-lactose or lactose-free diet or take lactase enzyme supplements.

Anemia

Children with classic CD are likely to have anemia or iron deficiency that is diagnosed via a complete blood cell count, an iron panel, and a ferritin test. If iron therapy is needed, the typical dose ranges between 2 and 5 mg of elementary iron per kilogram body weight. The dose depends on the severity of iron deficiency.

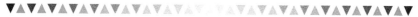

Osteopenia/Osteoporosis

A dual-energy x-ray absorptiometry (DEXA) scan is useful for children with classic symptoms of CD. Children with atypical symptoms are unlikely to have abnormal bone density. Nutritional counseling is indicated to ensure that patients have adequate calcium and vitamin D intake to prevent osteopenia and osteoporosis.

Transient Pancreatic Insufficiency

Patients with classic CD may have temporary pancreatic hypofunction. If the child does not gain sufficient weight on a strict GFD, then he or she may benefit from pancreatic enzyme supplementation to facilitate weight gain. The duration of enzyme therapy is usually 3 to 4 months (Evidence level III).

Lymphocytic Gastritis

Lymphocytic gastritis is reported in patients with CD. It usually resolves with a GFD and does not require other treatment unless the child has epigastric abdominal pain.

LONG-TERM MONITORING

The most likely cause of persistent symptoms is continued gluten ingestion, which can be voluntary or inadvertent. Other causes of nonresponsiveness are lactose malabsorption, unrecognized chronic giardiasis, food allergies (eg, milk, soy), and secondary pancreatic insufficiency in children. Newly diagnosed patients tend to develop constipation and fecal impaction because of the combined mucosal recovery and sudden dietary changes that may result in intermittent periumbilical pain.

Long-term monitoring of patients calls for periodic celiac serology tests, as well as an assessment of nutritional status and measurement of height, weight, and BMI (or weight for height ratio). In 2004, a consensus development conference convened by the National Institutes of Health developed a mnemonic for managing and monitoring patients with CD (**Box 4-5**).

Box 4-5. National Institutes of Health Mnemonic for the Management of Celiac Disease

C	Consultation with a skilled dietitian
E	Education about the disease
L	Lifelong adherence to a gluten-free diet
I	Identification and treatment of nutritional deficiencies
A	Access to an advocacy group
C	Continuous long-term follow-up by a multidisciplinary team

From NIH consensus statement on celiac disease. *NIH Consens State Sci Statements*. 2004; 21(1):1–22. https://consensus.nih.gov/2004/2004CeliacDisease118PDF.pdf. Accessed March 13, 2019.

SUGGESTED READING

Carroccio A, Iacono G, Montalto G, et al. Exocrine pancreatic function in children with coeliac disease before and after a gluten free diet. *Gut*. 1991;32(7):796–799

Fasano A, Berti I, Gerarduzzi T, et al. Prevalence of celiac disease in at-risk and not-at-risk groups in the United States: a large multicenter study. *Arch Intern Med*. 2003;163(3):286–292

Hill ID, Dirks MH, Liptak GS, et al; North American Society for Pediatric Gastroenterology, Hepatology and Nutrition. Guideline for the diagnosis and treatment of celiac disease in children: recommendations of the North American Society for Pediatric Gastroenterology, Hepatology and Nutrition. *J Pediatr Gastroenterol Nutr*. 2005,40(1):1–19

Hill ID, Fasano A, Guandalini S, et al. NASPGHAN clinical report on the diagnosis and treatment of gluten-related disorders. .*J Pediatr Gastroenterol Nutr*. 2016;63(1):156–165

Husby S, Koletzko S, Korponay-Szabó IR, et al; ESPGHAN Working Group on Coeliac Disease Diagnosis; ESPGHAN Gastroenterology Committee; European Society for Pediatric Gastroenterology, Hepatology, and Nutrition. European Society for Pediatric Gastroenterology, Hepatology, and Nutrition guidelines for the diagnosis of coeliac disease. *J Pediatr Gastroenterol Nutr*. 2012;54(1):136–160

Ludvigsson JF, Agreus L, Ciacci C, et al. Transition from childhood to adulthood in coeliac disease: the Prague consensus report. *Gut*. 2016;65(8):1242–1251

▼▲▼▲▼▲▼▲▼▲▼▲▼▲▼▲▼ ▼▲▼▲▼▲▼▲▼▲▼▲▼▲▼

Ludvigsson JF, Leffler DA, Bai JC, et al. The Oslo definitions for coeliac disease and related terms. *Gut.* 2013;62(1):43–52

National Institutes of Health Consensus Development Conference Statement on Celiac Disease, June 28-30, 2004. *Gastroenterology.* 2005;128(4 Suppl 1):S1–S9

Snyder J, Butzner JD, DeFelice AR, et al. Evidence-informed expert recommendations for the management of celiac disease in children. *Pediatrics.* 2016;138(3):e20153147

Constipation and Encopresis

Jason E. Dranove, MD

OVERVIEW

Up to 3% of visits to general pediatricians and 25% of visits to a pediatric gastroenterologist concern the issues of constipation and encopresis. Although parents commonly worry about a serious underlying condition, more than 95% of cases are considered *functional* (no identifiable metabolic, neurological, or anatomic cause) and require no significant workup. In most cases, a thorough history and physical examination are all that is needed to make a diagnosis (Evidence Level III). Formal definitions have been developed (**Box 5-1**).

Box 5-1. Definition of Functional Constipation

- Two of the following signs/symptoms present for at least 1 month
- Two or fewer defecations per week
- At least 1 episode of incontinence after the acquisition of toileting skills (infants and toddlers) or at least 1 episode of fecal incontinence per week (children 4–18 y)
- History of excessive stool retention
- Painful or hard bowel movements
- Presence of a large fecal mass in the rectum
- History of large-diameter stools that may obstruct the toilet

When constipation progresses to the point of a rectal fecal impaction, encopresis (the involuntary passage of stool) can ensue. A related but pathophysiologically separate condition exists in which the child beyond the toilet-training age (developmental age of at least 4 years) has fecal soiling in the absence of functional fecal retention. This condition is called nonretentive fecal incontinence.

Key facts to assist the clinician in identifying functional versus organic causes of constipation are as follows (Evidence Level III):

- Lack of a meconium bowel movement in the first 48 hours after birth warrants a mandatory investigation for Hirschsprung disease or anorectal malformations.
- Breastfed infants can stool as frequently as every feeding or as infrequently as every 10 to 14 days and still be considered healthy.
- Average stool frequency peaks in infancy at roughly 3 times per day and slows to roughly 1 time per day as the child approaches 1 year of age.
- Infants often appear to be constipated, to strain, and to have discomfort when passing stool. Passage of a soft bowel movement relieves the discomfort. This behavior is called infantile dyschezia and typically resolves by 9 months of age.
- Onset of functional constipation peaks at 3 times: transition from formula or human milk to cow's milk, toilet training, and the commencement of school.
- Nonretentive encopresis is often seen in the context of behavioral comorbidities or significant stress.

CAUSES

Functional constipation is the most common cause of constipation and encopresis in all age groups except the immediate newborn. The most well-accepted cause of constipation is that the child has a painful or an uncomfortable bowel movement and when further urges to defecate occur, the child consciously or unconsciously withholds stool by contracting the gluteal and pelvic muscles. Eventually, the rectum habituates to the stimulus of the enlarging fecal mass, the urge to defecate subsides, and a vicious cycle ensues.

Although children with behavioral and developmental challenges, such as attention-deficit/hyperactivity disorder, sensory integration dysfunction, and autism spectrum disorder, are at higher risk of developing constipation, they are generally included in the functional category, barring other findings. The differential diagnosis is shown in **Box 5-2**.

Box 5-2. Organic Causes of Constipation

Anatomic malformations
- Imperforate anus
- Anal stenosis
- Anteriorly displaced anus

Metabolic abnormalities
- Hypothyroidism
- Hypercalcemia
- Hypokalemia
- Cystic fibrosis
- Celiac disease

Neuropathic
- Myelomeningocele
- Spinal cord injury/ trauma
- Spinal dysraphism

Intestinal muscle/ nerve disorders
- Hirschsprung disease
- Internal anal sphincter achalasia
- Scleroderma
- Systemic lupus erythematosus
- Generalized hypotonia (eg, Down syndrome, muscular dystrophy)

Drugs
- Opiates
- Anticholinergics
- Phenobarbital

Other
- Lead intoxication
- Botulism
- Cow's milk protein intolerance
- History of sexual, physical, or emotional abuse

EVALUATION

History

Clues to functional constipation include the onset of constipation at common transitional times (ie, changing from formula or human milk to cow's milk, toilet training, or entering school) and parents' observance of voluntary stool withholding, such as leg straightening, gluteal clenching, standing with legs crossed in a hunched position, and disappearance of the child into another room during defecation times. The presence of small amounts of bright red blood on the outside of the stool or upon wiping likely indicates an anal fissure. Bright red blood consistently mixed in stool is more concerning for an underlying organic cause. Rectal prolapse can be seen in functional constipation, but recurrent prolapse without obvious constipation should prompt concern for cystic fibrosis.

Cow's milk allergy or intolerance is not a proven cause, but if intake is excessive, it might contribute to constipation by means of an unknown mechanism (Evidence Level III). Patients with fecal impactions frequently have urinary soiling secondary to bladder compression, which can lead to frequent urinary tract infections. Although no direct correlation has been proven, inadequate intake of clear liquids and low-fiber diets may contribute to constipation (Evidence Level III). The red flags on history that can indicate an underlying organic pathology are shown in **Table 5-1**.

Physical Examination

The abdominal examination findings in a patient with functional constipation can range from normal with no palpable stool to fullness with or without a palpable fecal impaction in the suprapubic and/or lower abdominal quadrants. No significant tenderness should be present. Additional physical examination findings for functional constipation include within–reference range growth parameters; normal lower-extremity deep tendon reflexes, strength, and gait; and normal cremasteric reflexes in boys. The clinician should perform a perianal examination to assess for anal position, injury, and fissure, as well as gluteal musculature. A digital rectal examination with the fifth finger should be performed in all constipated infants to assess sphincter tone and anal position (Evidence Level III). Rectal examination in older children is not mandatory if the physician is confident in the diagnosis. If a fecal impaction is suspected but not palpated on the abdominal examination, a digital rectal examination can be performed to confirm the diagnosis. The clinician should examine the lower back for signs of spinal dysraphism (eg, tuft of hair, deep dimple). The following red flag findings can easily be ascertained on physical examination (**Table 5-2**).

Laboratory Studies

Because most cases of functional constipation can be diagnosed based on history and physical examination findings, no workup is required (Evidence Level III). If the abdominal examination does not reveal an obvious fecal mass and a rectal examination is not performed, an abdominal radiograph can be helpful

Table 5-1. Historical Clues to Etiology of Constipation

Findings on History	Associated Conditions
Delayed passage of meconium	Hirschsprung disease Imperforate anus Small left colon Meconium ileus
Poor growth/heat or cold intolerance	Hypothyroidism
FTT, extraintestinal manifestations, abdominal distension, anemia, hypoalbuminemia	Celiac disease
Refractory urinary incontinence/recurrent UTI	Spinal cord abnormality
Acute-onset constipation	Sexual abuse Spinal cord injury/tumor
Recurrent respiratory tract infections and FTT, rectal prolapse	Cystic fibrosis
Honey ingestion in infant	Botulism
Sudden bloody diarrhea in a constipated infant	Hirschsprung enterocolitis
Lower-extremity weakness, numbness, tingling	Spinal cord abnormality
Developmental delay/hypotonia	Chromosomal abnormality Muscular dystrophies
Recurrent abdominal distension	Pseudo-obstruction Hirschsprung disease Recurrent sigmoid volvulus
Persistent bright red blood mixed in stool	Large polyp or obstructing mass
Fecal incontinence with no history of constipation	Nonretentive encopresis

Abbreviations: FTT, failure to thrive; UTI, urinary tract infection.

Table 5-2. Physical Examination Clues to Etiology of Constipation

Examination Finding	Condition Suggested
Short stature, coarse hair, macroglossia	Hypothyroidism
Sacral dimple, sacral tuft, absent DTR	Spina bifida (eg, myelomeningocele) Tethered spinal cord
Explosive stool upon finger withdrawal on rectal examination of infant	Hirschsprung disease
Absent or very small anal opening	Imperforate anus/anorectal malformation
Very tight anal canal of infant	Hirschsprung disease or anal stenosis
FTT, dermatitis herpetiformis, abdominal distension	Celiac disease
Hypotonia	Muscular dystrophy/SMA
Coarse lungs, fingernail clubbing, abdominal distension, rectal prolapse, FTT	Cystic fibrosis

Abbreviations: DTR, deep tendon reflexes; FTT, failure to thrive; SMA, spinal muscular atrophy.

(Evidence Level II-2). A workup is not indicated unless there are red flag findings on history or physical examination, or aggressive medical management and education have been unsuccessful. The North American Society for Pediatric Gastroenterology, Hepatology, and Nutrition has published an algorithm to guide physicians in the evaluation of constipation (**Figure 5-1**).

In children older than 1 year, the only screening tests recommended for refractory constipation are thyroid studies, a tissue transglutaminase IgA antibody level test, and a total serum IgA count (to rule out celiac disease) (Evidence Level III). A barium enema is not recommended to diagnose Hirschsprung disease, as the diagnosis can be missed by this modality. The only reliable methods of diagnosing Hirschsprung disease are by the absence of ganglion cells on an appropriate-depth rectal biopsy specimen or by lack of relaxation of the internal anal sphincter on an anorectal manometry (Evidence Level II-1). Cases truly refractory to medical management may require more in-depth testing (**Box 5-3**).

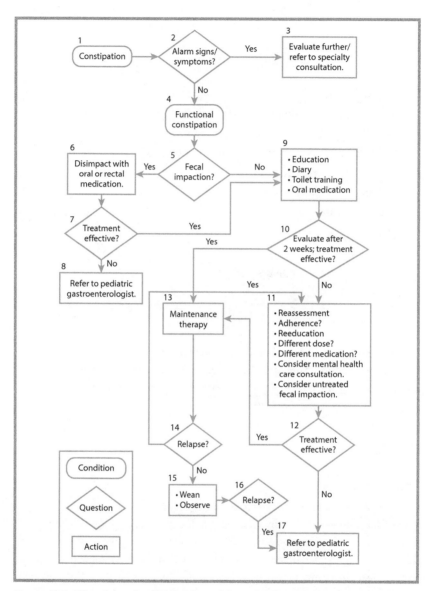

Figure 5-1. Algorithm for Evaluation of Constipation (Evidence Level III)

Abbreviations: exam, examination; MRI, magnetic resonance imaging; PEG, polyethylene glycol; psych, psychiatric; T4, anti-thyroxine; Rx, prescription; TSH, thyroid-stimulating hormone.

Modified with permission from Tabbers MM, DiLorenzo C, Berger MY, et al; European Society for Gastroenterology, Hepatology, and Nutrition; North American Society for Pediatric Gastroenterology. Evaluation and treatment of functional constipation in infants and children: evidence-based recommendations from ESPGHAN and NASPGHAN. *J Pediatr Gastroenterol Nutr.* 2014;58(2):258–274.

Box 5-3. Additional Testing at Subspecialty Level

Radiography
- Radiopaque marker transit study
- Barium enema
- Lumbosacral spine magnetic resonance imaging

Physiological testing
- Anorectal manometry
- Colonic manometry

Tissue sample
- Rectal suction biopsy
- Full-thickness rectal wall biopsy

Refractory constipation should not prompt a magnetic resonance imaging lumbar spine unless there are other concerning neurological symptoms (lower-extremity weakness, significant urinary incontinence, gait disturbances) or physical examination findings.

MANAGEMENT

Disimpaction

The key to successful management of constipation involves staged therapy, with disimpaction followed by maintenance therapy and ongoing education/behavioral modification. Disimpaction is not necessary in all cases; however, initiating maintenance therapy before disimpaction if a fecal impaction is present can lead to soiling, increased patient frustration, and distrust of medications. Clearing a fecal impaction will usually allow the rectum to decompress and regain sensation and tone.

Disimpaction can be accomplished via the oral, rectal, or combined route (Evidence Level II-3). In most cases, an initial trial of oral disimpaction with osmotic and occasionally stimulant laxatives is successful (Evidence Level II-3). Dosing varies by age and clinician, but most treating clinicians use

Box 5-4. Levine Children's Hospital 1-Day Bowel Cleanout

Age 1–2 y
- PEG 3350: 2 rounded teaspoons mixed in 4 oz of clear liquid hourly until stool is clear

Age 3–5 y
- PEG 3350: 4 capfuls mixed in 24 oz of clear liquid
- Give 4 oz every 30 minutes as tolerated; give 1 crushed tablet of bisacodyl 5 mg before and after PEG solution.

Age 6–11 y
- PEG 3350: 6–8 capfuls mixed in 24–48 oz of clear liquid
- Give 4 oz every 30 minutes as tolerated; give 1 tablet of bisacodyl before and after PEG solution.

Age 12 y and older
- PEG 3350: 8–10 capfuls mixed in 32–48 oz of clear liquid
- Give 4 oz every 30 minutes as tolerated; give 2 tablets of bisacodyl before and after PEG solution.

Sodium phosphate enema[a] administration (if needed)
- Age <2 y: not routinely recommended
- Age 2–4 y: 33.75 mL
- Age 5–11 y: 67.5 mL
- Age ≥12 y: 118 mL
- Give 1 bisacodyl tablet = 5 mg; give 1 capful of PEG 3350 = 17 g.

Abbreviation: PEG, polyethylene glycol.

[a] Sodium phosphate enema = monobasic sodium phosphate monohydrate 19 g and dibasic sodium phosphate heptahydrate 7 g/118 mL.

▼▲▼▲▼▲▼▲▼▲▼▲▼▲▼ ▼▲▼▲▼▲▼▲▼▲▼▲▼▲▼

polyethylene glycol 3350 (PEG 3350), an osmotic laxative, as the main component (**Box 5-4**).

Maintenance

In children without impaction, or after disimpaction is complete, maintenance
treatment is initiated. The goals of treatment are to achieve 1 to 2 soft stools a
day (a consistency of pudding or mashed potato), resolution of soiling, return of
rectal sensation, empowerment of the child, and removal of negative emotions
associated with the defecation process. Patients with mild cases might respond
to simple measures such as increased fiber in the diet, increased clear fluids,
and fruit juices with nonabsorbable sugars such as pear, prune, or apple juice
(Evidence Level II-3). Polyethylene glycol 3350 is the mainstay of treatment; it
is an osmotic laxative that helps soften and lubricate stool and is safe for use by
patients as young as 6 months (Evidence Level III). No serious adverse effects
from PEG 3350 have been confirmed; the most common adverse effects are diarrhea, bloating, and abdominal cramping, which usually can be managed with
dosing titration. Although PEG 3350 is likely safe for all ages, lactulose is the
recommended first-line treatment for infants younger than 6 months (Evidence
Level III). After infancy, stimulant laxatives may be used intermittently for
breakthrough constipation or if the symptoms are not responding adequately
to osmotic laxatives (Evidence Level II-1) (**Table 5-3**). Newer medications
lubiprostone and linaclotide are not recommended for the routine treatment of
functional constipation in children.

Education/Behavioral Modification

When dealing with constipation, education, continued reassurance, and positive
reinforcement are as important as medications. Attempting bowel movements
twice a day, after breakfast and dinner, helps the patient take advantage of the
gastrocolic reflex. Other strategies to consider include
- Eliminating distractions while in the bathroom (eg, electronic devices and
  games)
- Limiting attempts to 5 to 10 minutes (Longer attempts without a bowel
  movement can increase frustration and defiance.)
- Using techniques to increase the Valsalva maneuver, such as blowing up a
  balloon or blowing on the back of the hand
- Using a reasonable reward system, focusing on the positives and avoiding
  negative reinforcement
- Increasing intake of clear fluids, fiber, and fruit and vegetables (Although
  these nourishments are not scientifically proven to help, they are generally
  viewed as helpful.)

Table 5-3. Common Medications for Maintenance Treatment

Medication	Dose	Notes
Osmotic Laxatives		
Lactulose	10 g/15 mL liquid 1–3 mL/kg/d in 2 divided doses	Best for age <6 mo Can cause irritability because of flatulence and increased gas
Magnesium hydroxide	400 mg/5 mL 1–3 mL/kg/d	Should be used cautiously in infants
PEG 3350	One capful = 17 g 0.7–1.0 g/kg/d	Widespread use in infants not studied Should be mixed with clear liquid for best palatability
Stimulant Laxatives		
Senna	8.8 mg/5 mL 8.6-mg tablet 2–6 y: 2.5–7.5 mL/d >6 y: 1–3 tablets per day	Best used intermittently May be used as maintenance therapy in refractory cases
Bisacodyl	5-mg tablet (may be crushed) 3–11 y: 2.5–5 mg/dose >11 y: 5–10 mg/dose	Best used intermittently Use limited by adverse effects of cramping and abdominal pain

Abbreviation: PEG, polyethylene glycol.

Eliminating milk is not routinely recommended, although cutting back on excessive intake is reasonable. In general, if constipation starts during potty training, attempts at weaning therapy before achieving toileting independence are not advised, as hard or painful stools can impair progress in this endeavor.

LONG-TERM MONITORING

Laboratory or radiographic studies are not recommended routinely during treatment for constipation. Poorly controlled constipation over many years can result in quality of life impairment, social isolation, and family stress. In fact, up to 50% of patients experience a relapse within 2 years after an initial successful period (Evidence Level II-3). No official guidelines on treatment duration are available. A large study from Europe showed that up to 70% of patients were successfully treated 5 years after diagnosis, with most off of laxatives; therefore, the prognosis overall is positive (Evidence Level II-3).

SUGGESTED READING

Bongers EJ, Tabbers MM, Benninga MA. Functional nonretentive fecal incontinence in children. *J Pediatr Gastroenterol Nutr.* 2007;44(1):5–13

Kaugars A, Silverman A, Kinservik, et al. Families' perspectives on the effect of constipation and fecal incontinence on quality of life. *J Pediatr Gastroenterol Nutr.* 2010;51(6):747–752

Marloes EK, Bongers EJ, Van Wijk MP, Benninga MA. Long-term prognosis for childhood constipation: clinical outcomes in adulthood. *Pediatrics.* 2010;126(1):e156–e162

Michail S, Gendy E, Preud'Homme D, Mezoff A. Polyethylene glycol for constipation in children younger than eighteen months old. *J Pediatr Gastroenterol Nutr.* 2004;39(2):197–199

Pashankar DS, Bishop WP. Efficacy and optimal dose of daily polyethylene glycol 3350 for treatment of constipation and encopresis in children. *Pediatrics.* 2001;139(3):428–432

Pashankar DS, Loening-Baucke V, Bisohp WP. Safety of polyethylene glycol 3350 for the treatment of chronic constipation in children. *Arch Pediatr Adolesc Med.* 2003;157(7):661–664

Tabbers MM, DiLorenzo C, Berger MY, et al. Evaluation and treatment of functional constipation in infants and children: evidence-based guidelines from ESPGHAN and NASPGHAN. *J Pediatr Gastroenterol Nutr.* 2014;58(2):258–274

Diarrhea

Ricardo A. Caicedo, MD

OVERVIEW

Diarrhea is an increase in frequency or water content of stools resulting from an imbalance between intestinal water and electrolyte secretion and absorption. Expected stool frequency and volume vary by age (**Table 6-1**).

A more practical definition of diarrhea (except in breastfed infants) is the passage of liquid stools more than 3 times per day, or the passage of stools that are looser or more liquid than normal for the individual. *Acute diarrhea* in children usually is caused by infectious processes and typically has an onset and resolution within 1 to 2 weeks. When it is not self-limited and persists beyond this time frame, it is referred to as *chronic diarrhea.*

Table 6-1. Reference Range for Stool Frequency or Volume, by Age Group

Population	Reference Range for Stool Frequency or Volume
Breastfed infants	Once every 7 days to 7 times per day
Infants	5–10 g/kg/d
Children	0–3 stools per day, 10 mL/kg/d
Adolescents	0–2 stools per day, 200 g/d

CAUSES AND DIFFERENTIAL DIAGNOSIS

Most cases of acute diarrhea in infants and children are caused by a gastrointestinal (GI) infection (**Table 6-2**). In about two-thirds of cases, the infectious agent is identified. Viral causes are more common (50%–80%) and tend to present with watery diarrhea, and often with concomitant vomiting, as in acute gastroenteritis. Norovirus is now the leading cause of gastroenteritis in medical

Table 6-2. Causes of Acute Diarrhea

Gastrointestinal Infection

Viral	Bacterial	Protozoan
Rotavirus	Enteroinvasive *Escherichia coli*	*Giardia lamblia*
Norovirus	Enterohemorrhagic *E coli*	*Cryptosporidium parvum*
Enterovirus	Enterotoxigenic *E coli*	*Entamoeba histolytica*
Calicivirus	Enteropathogenic *E coli*	*Isospora belli*
Astrovirus	*Shigella* species	
	Salmonella species	
	Yersinia species	
	Campylobacter species	
	Clostridium difficile species	
	Vibrio cholerae species	
	Aeromonas species	

Nongastrointestinal Infection	Other
Influenza	Antibiotic associated
Otitis media	Drug adverse effect
Other respiratory tract infection	Food poisoning
Urinary tract infection	Allergic reaction
Meningitis	Acute appendicitis
Sepsis	Intussusception

▼▲▼▲▼▲▼▲▼▲▼▲▼▲▼ ▼ ▼ ▲▼▲▼▲▼▲▼▲▼▲▼▲▼

facilities in the United States, attributable to the widespread use of vaccination against rotavirus. Other etiologic categories for acute diarrhea include non-GI infection, toxin/drug, and allergy.

The differential diagnosis of prolonged or chronic diarrhea is much broader than that of acute diarrhea. Causes of chronic diarrhea can be categorized by mechanism (**Table 6-3**). Because many of these conditions appear primarily at specific ages, it also is helpful to stratify them by age at onset (**Table 6-4**).

In developing countries, chronic diarrhea is more likely to be caused by chronic parasitic (including helminths or worms), bacterial, or mycobacterial infection. Postinfectious villous injury and disaccharidase deficiency are also common. The most common causes of chronic diarrhea in industrialized nations are functional/dietary causes, carbohydrate malabsorption, celiac disease, and inflammatory bowel disease.

CLINICAL FEATURES

Acute diarrhea is frequently watery and often associated with nausea, vomiting, anorexia, cramping abdominal pain, and, in some cases, fever, fatigue, and generalized malaise. Blood and mucus in the stools in the acute scenario suggest infectious colitis. The term *dysentery* is often used to describe a syndrome of bloody diarrhea, tenesmus, and abdominal pain. Common infectious agents causing dysentery include *Salmonella, Shigella, Campylobacter*, and *Yersinia* species and enterohemorrhagic *Escherichia coli*. It is important to differentiate acute watery diarrhea from acute bloody diarrhea.

Recognizing dehydration caused by acute diarrhea is crucial, as it will dictate management decisions. The degree of dehydration is determined by stool volume, rapidity of onset, and duration of the diarrheal illness, as well as concomitant vomiting. Cardinal signs of dehydration include thirst, lack of tears, dry mucous membranes, decreased skin turgor, decreased urine output, and tachycardia.

The clinical picture in chronic diarrhea is more diverse. Stools may be watery, bloody, laden with mucus, oily, foamy, or explosive or they may contain undigested food particles. Parents typically observe and report the consistency and color of the stools. Red (blood), black (melena), or white (cholestasis) stools should prompt concern, but other hues including green and yellow can be within the reference range. Chronic diarrhea may lead to dehydration, but more commonly it affects nutrition and growth. In general, osmotic diarrhea (as seen with lactose intolerance) is associated with bloating and flatulence and improves with fasting. Voluminous diarrhea that persists in the fasting state implies a

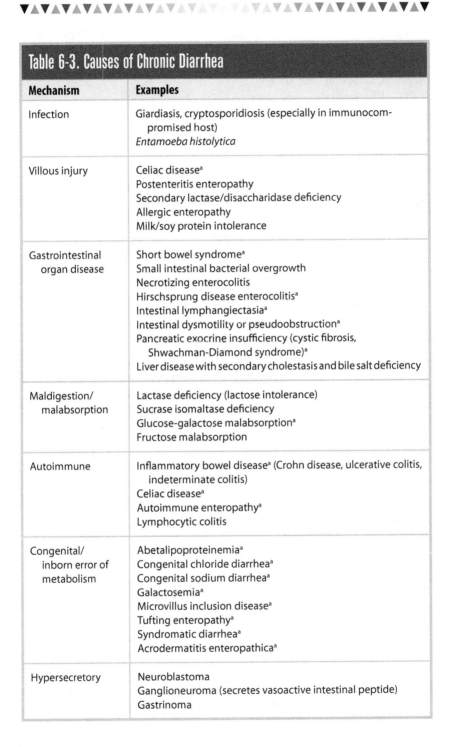

Table 6-3. Causes of Chronic Diarrhea

Mechanism	Examples
Infection	Giardiasis, cryptosporidiosis (especially in immunocompromised host) *Entamoeba histolytica*
Villous injury	Celiac disease[a] Postenteritis enteropathy Secondary lactase/disaccharidase deficiency Allergic enteropathy Milk/soy protein intolerance
Gastrointestinal organ disease	Short bowel syndrome[a] Small intestinal bacterial overgrowth Necrotizing enterocolitis Hirschsprung disease enterocolitis[a] Intestinal lymphangiectasia[a] Intestinal dysmotility or pseudoobstruction[a] Pancreatic exocrine insufficiency (cystic fibrosis, Shwachman-Diamond syndrome)[a] Liver disease with secondary cholestasis and bile salt deficiency
Maldigestion/ malabsorption	Lactase deficiency (lactose intolerance) Sucrase isomaltase deficiency Glucose-galactose malabsorption[a] Fructose malabsorption
Autoimmune	Inflammatory bowel disease[a] (Crohn disease, ulcerative colitis, indeterminate colitis) Celiac disease[a] Autoimmune enteropathy[a] Lymphocytic colitis
Congenital/ inborn error of metabolism	Abetalipoproteinemia[a] Congenital chloride diarrhea[a] Congenital sodium diarrhea[a] Galactosemia[a] Microvillus inclusion disease[a] Tufting enteropathy[a] Syndromatic diarrhea[a] Acrodermatitis enteropathica[a]
Hypersecretory	Neuroblastoma Ganglioneuroma (secretes vasoactive intestinal peptide) Gastrinoma

Table 6-3. Causes of Chronic Diarrhea (*continued*)

Mechanism	Examples
Hypermotility	Hyperthyroidism[a] Pseudo-obstruction[a] Short bowel syndrome[a]
Dietary/functional	Toddler's diarrhea (chronic nonspecific diarrhea of childhood) Hyperosmolar formula or juice Sorbitol Laxative overuse/abuse Encopresis (retentive fecal soiling) Irritable bowel syndrome

[a] Associated with poor weight gain, malnutrition, or failure to thrive.
Derived from Zella GC, Israel EJ. Chronic diarrhea in children. *Pediatr Rev.* 2012;33(5):207–218.

Table 6-4. Causes of Chronic Diarrhea, by Age at Onset

Infant	Child	Adolescent
Milk/soy protein intolerance	Postenteritis enteropathy	Irritable bowel syndrome
Postenteritis enteropathy	Toddler's diarrhea	Postenteritis enteropathy
Hyperosmolar formula	Irritable bowel syndrome	Lactose intolerance
Cystic fibrosis	Lactose intolerance	Inflammatory bowel disease
Celiac disease	Celiac disease	Celiac disease
Short bowel syndrome	Inflammatory bowel disease	*Rare:* Hyperthyroidism, laxative abuse
Rare: Congenital/inborn errors of metabolism, autoimmune enteropathy	Cystic fibrosis Encopresis *Rare:* Pseudo-obstruction, secretory tumor	

Derived from Zella GC, Israel EJ. Chronic diarrhea in children. *Pediatr Rev.* 2012;33(5):207–218.

secretory process, as in cholera or a catecholamine-secreting tumor. **Table 6-5** lists clinical features that are clues to particular diagnoses in chronic diarrhea.

EVALUATION

The initial history should consider the child's age and focus on onset, duration, and associated symptoms. Whether the diarrhea is acute or chronic should be apparent within the first few minutes of the encounter. In a patient with acute

Table 6-5. Clinical Manifestations of Chronic Diarrhea

Sign or Symptom	Suggested Diagnoses
Bloating/cramping	Lactose intolerance, IBS, giardiasis
Excessive flatus, explosive stools	Carbohydrate malabsorption
Oily/greasy stools (steatorrhea)	CF, celiac disease, Shwachman-Diamond syndrome
Bloody/mucous stools	IBD, allergic colitis
Undigested food particles in stool	Toddler's diarrhea (CNSD)
Watery, profuse stools, hypokalemia, alkalosis	Secretory tumor (VIPoma, neuroblastoma)
Nocturnal defecation	IBD
Recurrent abdominal pain	IBD, celiac disease, IBS
Pain relieved with defecation	IBS
Constipation/stool withholding	Encopresis, laxative overuse
Weight loss	Celiac disease, IBD, CF, hyperthyroidism
Growth failure/short stature	Celiac disease, IBD, CF
Normal growth	CNSD, overfeeding, fructose/sorbitol malabsorption
Anemia	IBD, celiac disease
Arthritis	IBD, celiac disease
Recurrent oral ulcers	IBD
Erythema nodosum	IBD
Dermatitis herpetiformis	Celiac disease
Abdominal distention, vomiting	Pseudo-obstruction, dysmotility

Abbreviations: CF, cystic fibrosis; CNSD, chronic nonspecific diarrhea; IBD, irritable bowel disease; IBS, irritable bowel syndrome.

diarrhea, the history should center on travel, food exposure, group child care, ill contacts, antibiotic exposure, and community outbreak. The physical examination should begin with rapid assessment of the degree of dehydration. Attention should be paid to thirst and tear production (ie, decreased) and also heart rate, blood pressure, skin turgor, and urine output. In many cases, a clinical diagnosis of a viral infection can be made without stool examination or other laboratory tests. Routine stool testing for bacterial, viral, or protozoan pathogens is not recommended in most cases of acute diarrhea (Evidence Level III). Exceptions include age younger than 3 months, toxic or septic appearance, high fever, bloody stools, a history of foreign travel, or a community outbreak.

In a child with chronic diarrhea, the physician should first determine the character of the stools and any associated symptoms that may provide diagnostic clues (see **Table 6-5**). As with other digestive complaints, "red flag" symptoms such as weight loss, nocturnal defecation, abdominal pain, and vomiting should prompt consideration of an underlying organic disease process. Dietary and family history is critically important. The physical examination should start with a review of the patient's growth parameters and nutritional status, including the body mass index in children and weight-for-length ratio in infants and toddlers. Depending on the initial differential diagnosis, several stool and laboratory tests may be useful; the results may prompt further diagnostic investigation (**Table 6-6**).

MANAGEMENT

Acute Diarrhea

Treatment of acute diarrhea is directed toward maintaining hydration. Most patients have mild-to-moderate dehydration, and the first-line recommended treatment is oral rehydration. Glucose-electrolyte oral rehydration solutions enhance intestinal absorption of salt and water, and they can relatively rapidly (3–4 hours) rehydrate a child. If the child is unable to drink, the solution can be given via a nasogastric tube. Intravenous rehydration is indicated in patients with excessive vomiting, ongoing losses, or severe dehydration. Once rehydrated, the infant or child should resume an age-appropriate normal diet, which reduces intestinal permeability as well as protein and energy deficits (Evidence Level I). The popular BRAT (bananas, rice, applesauce, toast) diet is nutritionally inadequate and, thus, not recommended. Breastfed infants should continue to breastfeed at all times, including during rehydration. Use of diluted formula is not indicated.

Most cases of diarrhea caused by a GI infection do not require antimicrobial therapy. In patients with enterohemorrhagic *Escherichia coli*, for example,

Table 6-6. Diagnostic Tests in the Evaluation of Chronic Diarrhea

Test	Use/Implication
Stool	
Lactoferrin level/white blood cell count	Colonic inflammation (nonspecific cause)
Bacterial culture	Infectious enterocolitis
Clostridium difficile toxin assay	*C difficile* infection
Giardia/cryptosporidium antigen level	Specific protozoan infection
Presence of ova and parasites	*Entamoeba histolytica, Cyclospora,* helminths
pH/reducing substances	Carbohydrate malabsorption
Fat stain	Fat malabsorption
72-hour fecal fat collection	Evaluation of steatorrhea
Elastase (pancreatic elastase-1) level	Pancreatic exocrine insufficiency (low)
Alpha1-antitrypsin level	GI protein loss (high)
Osmotic gap $[290 - 2 \times (Na + K)]$	Classification of watery diarrhea (secretory vs osmotic)
Blood	
CBC/differential	Anemia in IBD, celiac disease, thrombocytosis, leukocytosis in IBD
ESR, C-reactive protein concentration	Elevated in IBD
Electrolyte level	Deranged in hypersecretory processes (hypokalemia, hyponatremia)
Albumin level	Low in IBD, protein-losing enteropathy
Total/direct bilirubin level	Cholestasis, CF
Tissue transglutaminase IgA titer	Celiac disease—first-line screening test[a] (Evidence Level I)
Vitamin A, D, and E levels	Fat malabsorption (CF, IBD, celiac disease)

Table 6-6. Diagnostic Tests in the Evaluation of Chronic Diarrhea (*continued*)

Test	Use/Implication
Blood (*continued*)	
Cholesterol, triglycerides levels	Low in abetalipoproteinemia
Other	
Sweat chloride	CF
Breath hydrogen testing	Carbohydrate malabsorption, small intestinal bacterial overgrowth
Abdominal radiograph	Fecal impaction, encopresis
Small bowel follow-through	Dysmotility, Crohn disease
EGD with biopsies	Celiac disease,[a] IBD,[a] disaccharidase deficiency
Pancreatic enzyme analysis	Pancreatic exocrine insufficiency
Colonoscopy with biopsies	IBD,[a] allergic colitis, lymphocytic colitis
Anorectal manometry/rectal biopsies	Hirschsprung disease

Abbreviations: CBC, complete blood cell count; CF, cystic fibrosis; EGD, esophagogastroduodenoscopy; ESR, erythrocyte sedimentation rate; IBD, irritable bowel disease; IBS, irritable bowel syndrome; K, potassium; Na, sodium.

[a] Evidence Level I.

antibiotics are contraindicated because they may increase the risk of developing hemolytic uremic syndrome. Antimicrobial therapy is recommended in the following infectious scenarios:

- *Salmonella typhi*
- *Salmonella* species in infants, sickle cell disease, immunocompromise (Evidence Level III)
- *Shigella* species (Evidence Level I)
- *Campylobacter* species (for severe cases) (Evidence Level II-3)
- Cholera (Evidence Level I)
- *Clostridium difficile* (metronidazole as first-line treatment, with oral vancomycin for recurrent or severe disease) (Evidence Level I)
- *Giardia* species (Evidence Level I), *Cryptosporidium* species, *Entamoeba histolytica*

Probiotics, live active microorganisms with a beneficial effect on the host, may be useful in certain cases of acute diarrhea such as rotaviral diarrhea, the duration and severity of which can be reduced with Lactobacillus rhamnosus GG (Evidence Level I). Probiotic preparations also have been shown to reduce the severity of antibiotic-associated diarrhea (Evidence Level I); however, the same effect has not been observed in bacterial infectious diarrhea.

The World Health Organization recommends zinc supplementation for the treatment of diarrhea in children 6 months and older. To date, the mechanism is undetermined, but benefit has been shown in patients in areas that have a high prevalence of zinc deficiency and malnutrition (Evidence Level I). Antimotility agents such as loperamide or diphenoxylate have no role in treating acute diarrhea, and their use may protract an acute infectious process or lead to ileus.

Chronic Diarrhea

Treatment of chronic diarrhea is specific to the underlying cause (**Table 6-7**). Furthermore, enteral or parenteral nutritional support may be needed in cases involving undernutrition or failure to thrive. Attention to weigh velocity and anthropometric measurements is essential to the management of chronic diarrhea.

LONG-TERM MONITORING

In many cases of chronic diarrhea, identification and treatment of the underlying cause leads to resolution of symptoms and prevents nutritional deficiencies. Patients on a low-lactose diet for lactose intolerance may require alternative sources of calcium to meet recommended targets. Patients with inflammatory bowel disease, celiac disease, cystic fibrosis, or short bowel syndrome should undergo longitudinal follow-up with specialists in gastroenterology and nutrition (Evidence Level III). Such follow-up also pertains to any infant or child receiving home parenteral nutrition or being evaluated for intestinal transplantation. These children will benefit from careful serial monitoring of weight velocity, linear growth, dietary intake, stooling pattern, blood counts, inflammatory markers (or tissue transglutaminase level in the case of celiac disease), protein status, and micronutrients/vitamins.

Table 6-7. Treatment of Chronic Diarrhea by Diagnosis

Diagnosis	Treatment
Allergic enteropathy	Protein hydrolysate or elemental formula
Autoimmune enteropathy	Immunosuppression
Bile acid malabsorption	Cholestyramine
Celiac disease	Gluten-free diet (Evidence Level I)
Chronic nonspecific diarrhea (toddler's diarrhea)	Reduce fructose/carbohydrate intake, liberalize fat, fiber
Congenital/neonatal diarrheas (microvillus inclusion disease, tufting enteropathy, congenital chloride, or sodium diarrhea)	Parenteral nutrition, aggressive fluid/ electrolyte replacement, intestinal transplantation
Cystic fibrosis	Pancreatic enzyme supplementation, enteral nutrition, fat-soluble vitamins
Giardiasis	Metronidazole (Evidence Level I), nitazoxanide
Glucose-galactose malabsorption	Fructose-based formula/diet (Evidence Level II-1)
Hirschsprung disease (enterocolitis)	Antibiotics, surgery
Inflammatory bowel disease	Immunosuppression, immunomodulation (Evidence Level I), enteral nutrition, biologics (Evidence Level I), antibiotics, surgery
Irritable bowel syndrome	Dietary modification, stress reduction, fiber (Evidence Level III), antimotility agents, antispasmodics
Lactose/fructose intolerance	Lactose/fructose-limited diet, lactase
Secretory diarrheas	Fluid/electrolyte replacement, parenteral nutrition, octreotide, racecadotril
Short bowel syndrome	Enteral and parenteral nutrition, loperamide, bowel-lengthening surgery, intestinal transplantation
Small intestinal bacterial overgrowth	Antibiotics (metronidazole, rifaximin) (Evidence Level II-1)
Sucrase-isomaltase deficiency	Dietary restriction, sacrosidase (Evidence Level I)

SUGGESTED READING

Armon K, Stephenson T, MacFaul R, Eccleston P, Werneke U. An evidence and consensus based guideline for acute diarrhoea management. *Arch Dis Child.* 2001;85(2):132–142

Binder HJ. Causes of chronic diarrhea. *N Engl J Med.* 2006;355(3):236–239

CaJacob NJ, Cohen MB. Update on diarrhea. *Pediatr Rev.* 2016;37(8):313–322

Davidson G, Barnes G, Bass D, et al. Infectious diarrhea in children: Working Group Report of the First World Congress of Pediatric Gastroenterology, Hepatology, and Nutrition. *J Pediatr Gastroenterol Nutr.* 2002;35(Suppl 2):S143–S150

Hempel S, Newberry SJ, Maher AR, et al. Probiotics for the prevention and treatment of antibiotic-associated diarrhea: a systematic review and meta-analysis. *JAMA.* 2012;307(18): 1959–1969

Hill ID, Dirks MH, Liptak GS, et al; North American Society for Pediatric Gastroenterology, Hepatology and Nutrition. Guideline for the diagnosis and treatment of celiac disease in children: recommendations of the North American Society for Pediatric Gastroenterology, Hepatology and Nutrition. *J Pediatr Gastroenterol Nutr.* 2005;40(1):1–19

King CK, Glass R, Bresee JS, Duggan C; Centers for Disease Control and Prevention. Managing acute gastroenteritis among children: oral rehydration, maintenance, and nutritional therapy. *MMWR Recommend Rep.* 2003;52(RR-16):1–16

Lazzerini M, Ronfani L. Oral zinc for treating diarrhoea in children. *Cochrane Database Syst Rev.* 2008;3:CD005436

Zella GC, Israel EJ. Chronic diarrhea in children. *Pediatr Rev.* 2012;33(5):207–218

Eosinophilic Esophagitis

Ameesh A. Shah, MD

OVERVIEW

Eosinophilic esophagitis (EoE) is a chronic, allergic inflammatory disease of the esophagus. The exact etiology is unknown, but EoE is thought to be triggered by an abnormal immunologic response to food antigens in the diet. Other potential causes are noted in **Box 7-1.** This disease can present with a wide variety of gastrointestinal symptoms depending on age and severity. Controversy exists regarding the optimal management and follow-up of this disease because the natural history is still under investigation.

SIGNS AND SYMPTOMS

Symptoms of EoE can vary greatly depending on the age of the child (**Box 7-2**).

Box 7-1. Causes of Esophageal Eosinophilia

- Gastroesophageal reflux disease
- Crohn disease
- Celiac disease
- Infection
- Connective tissue disease
- Graft-versus-host disease
- Drug hypersensitivity
- Eosinophilic gastroenteritis
- Pill-induced esophagitis

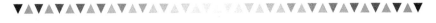

Box 7-2. Presentation of Symptoms by Age

Infants/toddlers
- Vomiting, feeding difficulties, poor weight gain

Children
- Abdominal/epigastric pain, dysphagia, poor appetite, choking

Adolescents
- Dysphagia, food impaction, reflux symptoms refractory to medical therapy

Vomiting and Feeding Difficulty

Infants and toddlers often present with vomiting and feeding difficulty. Vomiting is commonly seen with infantile reflux in the first 6 months after birth. Persistent or worsening symptoms that do not respond to acid suppression medications indicate the possibility of EoE rather than gastroesophageal reflux, which typically starts to improve when infants are 6 months of age. In some cases, EoE symptoms will improve with proton pump inhibitor (PPI) therapy. Vomiting related to EoE is usually associated with irritability and feeding difficulties such as choking, gagging, feeding refusal, or retching. Infants and toddlers with persistent feeding difficulties should be evaluated for EoE and treated to prevent poor weight gain and failure to thrive.

Dysphagia

Dysphagia is the most common symptom of EoE in school-aged children and teenagers. Children often report that food gets stuck in their throat or chest or that food feels like it's going down slowly. These symptoms can be intermittent and, therefore, are not reported promptly. Many patients have learned to overcome their symptoms by eating more slowly, chewing food into smaller pieces, drinking more while eating, and avoiding foods of certain consistencies, such as meats and bread, that may tend to get stuck. Food impaction is a common presenting symptom in EoE and may require endoscopic removal of the food bolus. Patients often report that they had had intermittent dysphagia for years before experiencing an episode of food impaction, but they attributed this to poor chewing or eating too quickly. Multiple biopsy specimens from the esophagus should always be obtained during endoscopic removal of an object or a food bolus.

Dysphagia and food impaction can result from a mechanical obstruction of the esophagus, which can be visualized by endoscopy or radiographically. It is unclear whether a focal stricture, concentric ring, or narrowed segment of the esophageal lumen is secondary to the degree of superficial inflammation, duration of disease, or involvement of deeper layers of the esophageal wall.

Pain

Pain is another common symptom of EoE, particularly in younger children who may not be able to accurately describe dysphagia. Epigastric, chest, and/or abdominal pain is often reported and can be intermittent in nature. This complaint should be investigated, especially when it is associated with other symptoms such as vomiting and poor weight gain and a history of other allergic conditions.

Allergies

The EoE population is highly atopic, with more than two-thirds of patients having another allergic disease such as asthma, eczema, food allergies, or environmental allergies. There seems to be a male predilection in both children and adults, and the disease is also more common in white patients. Regarding the age profile, the diagnosis is more common in the 5- to 10-year-old age group. As more adults are diagnosed, a familial pattern also has been observed, which may be related to the strong familial association with allergic diseases.

EVALUATION

Patients who have symptoms consistent with EoE should undergo an upper endoscopy with biopsies as the initial diagnostic step (**Figure 7-1**). Although visual findings such as mucosal edema and inflammation of the esophageal lining are typical, a small percentage of pediatric patients may have a normal-appearing esophagus during an endoscopy.

Obtaining multiple esophageal biopsy specimens during an endoscopy is essential in making the diagnosis. Because eosinophils are not typically found in the esophageal epithelium, their presence needs to be investigated. To receive a diagnosis of EoE, the patient should have clinical signs of esophageal dysfunction and eosinophilic infiltration of esophageal mucosa with at least 15 eosinophils in 1 high-power field. The eosinophilia must be isolated to the

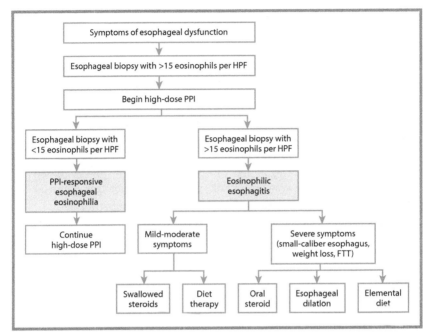

Figure 7-1. Diagnostic and Therapeutic Approach for Patients With Eosinophilic Esophagitis

Abbreviations: FTT, failure to thrive; HPF, high-power field; PPI, proton pump inhibitor therapy. Reproduced with permission from Ruffner MA, Spergel JM. Eosinophilic esophagitis in children. *Curr Allergy Asthma Rep*. 2017;17(8):54.

esophagus, and other causes of esophageal eosinophilia should be excluded (Evidence Level III).

Patients who have severe dysphagia may also benefit from an esophagram to identify the presence of a stricture and the need for therapeutic dilation. An upper-gastrointestinal series can also be ordered if vomiting is a predominant symptom.

MANAGEMENT

Medical

Corticosteroids are the most common medical intervention used in the treatment of EoE. Because of the decreased risk of adverse effects, topical steroids have become the preferred method over systemic steroids, as studies have demonstrated that they are equally effective in inducing histologic and symptomatic

▼▲▼▲▼▲▼▲▼▲▼▲▼▲▼ ▲▼▲▼▲▼▲▼▲▼▲▼▲▼▲▼

remission. Topical steroids can be administered via a puff-and-swallow mechanism using a metered dose inhaler of fluticasone at a dose of 2 puffs twice daily
(110-mcg dose inhaler for patients younger than 10 years or a 220-mcg dose
inhaler for those 10 years and older). This method of treatment has demonstrated a response rate of more than 50% in pediatric EoE (Evidence Level I).
Because young children or patients with developmental delay may be unable
to effectively use an inhaler device or display the appropriate swallow tech-
nique, a viscous solution of budesonide mixed with sucralose or honey also can
be used as treatment. Both adult and pediatric studies have found this method
to be effective, and it may be even more effective than fluticasone in achieving
histologic remission (Evidence Level II-1). Because EoE is a chronic disease,
there is a tendency for recurrences after topical steroid treatment is discon-
tinued, so most patients will continue taking budesonide and/or fluticasone as
maintenance therapy.

Proton pump inhibitors are now considered to be an option for first-line
therapy for EoE. Initially, PPIs were thought to be effective only in treating EoE
related to gastroesophageal reflux disease (GERD), but studies have shown that
even patients who do not have GERD achieve clinical and histologic resolution
of EoE with this treatment. Proton pump inhibitors seem to have multiple
anti-inflammatory effects in addition to antisecretory effects, which can prevent
recruitment of eosinophils to the esophageal mucosa.

Dietary

A link exists between food antigens in the diet and EoE. Because EoE is
thought to be caused by food, the identification and exclusion of trigger food(s)
is a possible treatment plan. An empiric elimination diet such as the Four Food
Elimination Diet removes the 4 most common foods implicated in EoE (milk,
wheat, egg, soy) from the patient's diet for at least 6 weeks. Allergy-directed
elimination diets based on skin prick testing and atopy patch testing have
also been used, but this approach has not been shown to be very helpful and
is falling out of favor. An exclusive amino-acid–based elemental formula is a
dietary therapy that has been shown to be most effective in inducing clinical
and histologic remission, but it is difficult to follow and maintain.

Esophageal Dilation

Esophageal dilation may be needed in patients who have esophageal narrowing
or strictures and who have not responded to medical or dietary treatment. This
treatment improves dysphagia and decreases episodes of food impaction in
a majority of patients with a reduced-caliber esophagus, but it does not treat

esophageal inflammation. Overall, endoscopic dilation is a safe procedure, with minimal risks or adverse events.

LONG-TERM MONITORING

Eosinophilic esophagitis tends to be a chronic inflammatory disease, but questions remain regarding diagnosis, treatment, and the natural history of the disorder. In addition, controversy exists surrounding the treatment of asymptomatic patients with esophageal eosinophilia. Esophageal strictures and small-caliber esophagus have been the major complications of untreated disease. Noninvasive testing is needed to reduce the number of endoscopies required to follow the disease and monitor patients' response to treatment. Fortunately, esophageal metaplasia has not been reported, even in patients with severe disease.

SUGGESTED READING

Cheng E, Zhang X, et al. Omeprazole blocks eotaxin-3 expression by oesophageal squamous cells from patients with eosinophilic oesophagitis and GORD. *Gut*. 2013;62(6):824–832

Gonsalves N, Yang GY, Doerfler B. Elimination diet effectively treats eosinophilic esophagitis in adults; food reintroduction identifies causative factors. *Gastroenterology*. 2012;142(7):141–149

Kagalwalla AF, Shah A, Li BU, et al. Identification of specific foods responsible for inflammation in children with eosinophilic esophagitis successfully treated with empiric elimination diet. *J Pediatr Gastroenterol Nutr*. 2011;53(2):145–149

Kim HP, Dellon ES. An evolving approach to the diagnosis of eosinophilic esophagitis. *Gastroenterol Hepatol*. 2018;14(6):358–366

Liacouras CA, Furuta GT, Hirano I, et al. Eosinophilic esophagitis: updated consensus recommendations for children and adults. *J Allergy Clin Immunol*. 2011;128(1):3–20

Lucendo AJ, Molina-Infante J, Aria A, et al. Guidelines on eosinophilic esophagitis: evidence based-statements and recommendations for diagnosis and management in children and adults. *United European Gastroenterol J*. 2017;5(3):335–358

Spergel JM, Brown-Whitehorn TF, Beausoliel JL, et al. 14 years of eosinophilic esophagitis: clinical features and prognosis. *J Pediatr Gastroenterol Nutr*. 2008;48(1):30–36

Straumann A, Aceves SS, Blanchard C, et al. Pediatric and adult eosinophilic esophagitis: similarities and differences. *Allergy*. 2012;67(4):477–490

Gastroesophageal Reflux

Neetu Bali, MD, MPH; Maya Gharfeh, MD, MPH;
Peter L. Lu, MD, MS; and Hayat Mousa, MD

DEFINITION

Gastroesophageal reflux (GER) is characterized by the passage of gastric contents into the esophagus with or without regurgitation or vomiting. This physiologic process occurs daily in healthy infants and children. Although this is a physiologic and often benign phenomenon, GER may evolve into gastro-esophageal reflux disease (GERD), with consistent histologic findings as well as complications, including failure to thrive, respiratory conditions, or swallowing disorders. Recent practice guidelines from the North American and European societies for pediatric gastroenterology define GERD as bothersome symptoms or complications related to GER.

CAUSES

Several barriers keep gastric contents in the stomach and prevent regurgitation and vomiting. The primary barriers are the lower esophageal sphincter (LES), the diaphragmatic pinchcock, and the angle of His. These barriers work together to limit the frequency and volume of refluxed gastric contents into the esophagus. The second line of defense is esophageal clearance, which is responsible for limiting the duration of contact between contents in the esophageal lumen and the esophageal epithelium. Finally, the third layer of protection involves salivary and esophageal secretions that work to neutralize the pH of the contents in the esophageal lumen. These barriers work in concert to minimize GER and GERD.

Gastroesophageal reflux can be categorized as primary or secondary. Primary GER results from abnormalities inherent to the upper gastrointestinal tract. Secondary GER results from abnormalities related to systemic disorders, neurologic disease, metabolic disorders, or various medications. Both primary and secondary GER arise from inappropriate relaxation of the LES and impaired esophageal clearance. GER evolves into GERD when protective measures of the esophagus fail to function appropriately, leading to increased reflux of gastric contents into the esophagus; poor clearance of the refluxed matter; and recurrent, bothersome symptoms such as emesis, pain, irritability, or feeding refusal. Given this difference, it is important to distinguish GER from GERD by means of a thorough clinical history and physical examination.

DIFFERENTIAL DIAGNOSIS

Differentiating GERD from other disorders based on clinical presentation alone can be challenging, and it is important to recognize symptoms and signs that suggest another etiology. The differential diagnosis for children with symptoms suggestive of GERD is extensive. Gastrointestinal disorders that can present in a similar manner include eosinophilic esophagitis, food allergy or intolerance, peptic ulcer disease, esophageal achalasia, gastroparesis, pancreatitis, inflammatory bowel disease, and a variety of conditions that can lead to gastrointestinal obstruction such as pyloric stenosis. In addition, nongastrointestinal causes, including neurologic, metabolic, endocrine, cardiac, infectious, renal, and behavioral conditions, should be considered in the appropriate clinical setting. Important aspects of the clinical presentation include the nature of the emesis, temporal relationship of the emesis with feeding, presence of bile or blood, forceful or projectile nature of the emesis, irritability with emesis, and fever or lethargy. The physician also should establish a thorough feeding history, including any dysphagia, food sticking, slow eating pace, and avoidance of certain foods, which may indicate eosinophilic esophagitis. In reviewing the child's medical history, the physician should note prematurity, neurologic disease, allergic conditions, growth or developmental delays, psychological conditions, and previous surgeries.

SIGNS AND SYMPTOMS

Infants

Physiological GER rarely begins before the age of 1 week or after the age of 6 months. Vomiting and regurgitation, or spitting up, are often nonspecific symptoms of GERD in infants. Presenting symptoms also can include irritability, dystonic neck posturing (Sandifer syndrome), feeding refusal, failure to thrive, aspiration, and potential apnea (**Table 8-1**). Obtaining a detailed feeding and dietary history is particularly important in infants; it should include the length of the feeding period, volume of each feed, quality of milk supply when

Table 8-1. Symptoms and Signs Associated With Gastroesophageal Reflux Disease in Infants and Children

Symptoms	Signs
General	
Discomfort/irritability[a]	Dental erosion
Failure to thrive	Anemia
Feeding refusal	
Dystonic neck posturing (Sandifer syndrome)	
Gastrointestinal	
Recurrent regurgitation with/without vomiting in the older child	Esophagitis
Heartburn/chest pain[b]	Esophageal stricture
Epigastric pain[b]	Barrett esophagus
Hematemesis	
Dysphagia/odynophagia	
Airway	
Wheezing	Apnea spells
Stridor	Asthma
Cough	Recurrent pneumonia associated with aspiration
Hoarseness	Recurrent otitis media

[a] If excessive discomfort/irritability and pain are the only manifestations, it is unlikely to be related to gastroesophageal reflux disease.

[b] Typical symptoms of gastroesophageal reflux disease in older children.

Adapted with permission from Rosen R, Vandenplas Y, Singendonk M, et al. Pediatric gastroesophageal reflux clinical practice guidelines: joint recommendations of the North American Society for Pediatric Gastroenterology, Hepatology, and Nutrition and the European Society for Pediatric Gastroenterology, Hepatology, and Nutrition. *J Pediatr Gastroenterol Nutr.* 2018;66(3):516–554.

▼▲▼▲▼▲▼▲▼▲▼▲▼▲▼   ▼▲▼▲▼▲▼▲▼▲▼▲▼▲▼

breastfeeding, type of formula, methods of mixing the formula, food additives, restriction of allergens, and interval between feedings. In addition, the physician should obtain a detailed history of the infant's pattern of regurgitation or vomiting, including any nocturnal emesis, the length of time after meals that these events occur, whether emesis is digested or undigested, and any concern regarding bilious emesis.

Children and Adolescents

Symptoms of GERD in children and adolescents include regurgitation, vomiting, abdominal pain, and cough. Cough and feeding refusal are the most common presenting symptoms in children aged 1 to 5 years. Heartburn, abdominal pain, chest pain, nausea, and vomiting are the most common presenting symptoms of GERD in older children. It is important to recognize any red flag symptoms or signs that suggest disorders other than GERD (**Table 8-2**).

Table 8-2. Red Flag Symptoms and Signs That Suggest Disorders Other Than Gastroesophageal Reflux Disease in Infants and Children

Symptoms and Signs	Remarks
General	
Weight loss	Suggesting a variety of conditions, including systemic infections
Lethargy	
Excessive irritability/pain	
Dysuria	May suggest urinary tract infection, especially in infants and young children
Onset of regurgitation/ vomiting >6 months or increasing/persisting >12–18 months of age	Late onset as well as symptoms increasing or persisting after infancy, based on natural course of the disease, may indicate a diagnosis other than GERD
Neurological	
Bulging fontanel/rapidly increasing head circumference	May suggest raised intracranial pressure, for example, caused by meningitis, brain tumor, or hydrocephalus

Table 8-2. Red Flag Symptoms and Signs That Suggest Disorders Other Than Gastroesophageal Reflux Disease in Infants and Children (*continued*)

Symptoms and Signs	Remarks
Neurological (*continued*)	
Seizures	
Macro/microcephaly	
Gastrointestinal	
Persistent, forceful vomiting	Indicative of hypertrophic pyloric stenosis (infants up to 2 months old)
Nocturnal vomiting	May suggest increased intracranial pressure
Bilious vomiting	Regarded as symptom of intestinal obstruction; possible causes include Hirschsprung disease, intestinal atresia, or mid-gut volvulus or intussusception
Hematemesis	Suggests a potentially serious bleed from the esophagus, stomach, or upper gut, possibly GERD-associated, occurring from acid-peptic disease[a], Mallory-Weiss tear[b], or reflux-esophagitis
Chronic diarrhea	May suggest food protein-induced gastroenteropathy[c]
Rectal bleeding	Indicative of multiple conditions, including bacterial gastroenteritis, inflammatory bowel disease, as well as acute surgical conditions and food protein-induced gastroenteropathy rectal bleeding[c] (bleeding caused by proctocolitis)
Abdominal distension	Indicative of obstruction, dysmotility, or anatomic abnormalities

Abbreviations: GERD, gastroesophageal reflux disease; NSAID, nonsteroidal anti-inflammatory drugs.
[a] Especially with NSAID use.
[b] Associated with vomiting.
[c] More likely in infants with eczema and/or a strong family history of atopic disease.

Reproduced with permission from Rosen R, Vandenplas Y, Singendonk M, et al. Pediatric gastroesophageal reflux clinical practice guidelines: joint recommendations of the North American Society for Pediatric Gastroenterology, Hepatology, and Nutrition and the European Society for Pediatric Gastroenterology, Hepatology, and Nutrition. *J Pediatr Gastroenterol Nutr.* 2018;66(3):516–554.

▼▲▼▲▼▲▼▲▼▲▼▲▼▲▼▲   ▼▲▼▲▼▲▼▲▼▲▼▲▼▲▼

EVALUATION

For many patients, particularly older children who are developmentally normal, a comprehensive clinical history and physical examination can be sufficient to diagnose GERD. No single gold standard investigation exists to diagnose GERD in infants or children (Evidence Level III). Diagnostic studies can be used to document evidence of GERD, establish a temporal relationship between reflux events and symptoms, assess the patient's response to treatment, and exclude other diseases that may present in a manner similar to GERD. In the absence of concerning symptoms or signs, diagnostic testing or therapies are not recommended if the child's symptoms have no impact on feeding, growth, or attainment of developmental milestones. Guidelines for the evaluation and management of infants, children, and adolescents with suspected GER and GERD are shown in **figures 8-1** and **8-2**.

Multichannel Intraluminal Impedance and pH Monitoring

Multichannel intraluminal impedance (MII) monitoring records the presence of solids, fluids, and air in the esophagus based on changes in electrical impedance. It can distinguish between anterograde and retrograde movement and, thus, differentiate between a swallowed bolus and a reflux event. Multichannel intraluminal impedance is often combined with pH monitoring, which is used to differentiate acidic from nonacidic reflux events. An episode of reflux with a pH below 4.0 is considered an acidic reflux event.

Combined MII and pH monitoring is clinically indicated for patients with intractable symptoms such as chest or abdominal pain, apparent life-threatening events, apnea, choking, and stridor, particularly when the patient has not responded to initial medical treatment (Evidence Level III). Combining MII and pH monitoring can help in detecting refluxate with pH lower than 4 and greater than 4, full column refluxate, liquid and gas reflux, and declines in esophageal pH due to reflux versus swallow-related declines. However, the monitoring results may be difficult to interpret in patients with motility disorders, severe esophagitis, or other concurrent conditions.

Esophagogastroduodenoscopy

Signs or complications of GERD, including esophagitis, mucosal erosions, ulcers, and strictures, can be detected by endoscopy with biopsy. When the clinical diagnosis of GERD is in question, endoscopy with biopsy is indicated to rule out conditions that cause symptoms similar to those of GERD, such as eosinophilic esophagitis, esophageal stricture, infectious esophagitis, or Crohn

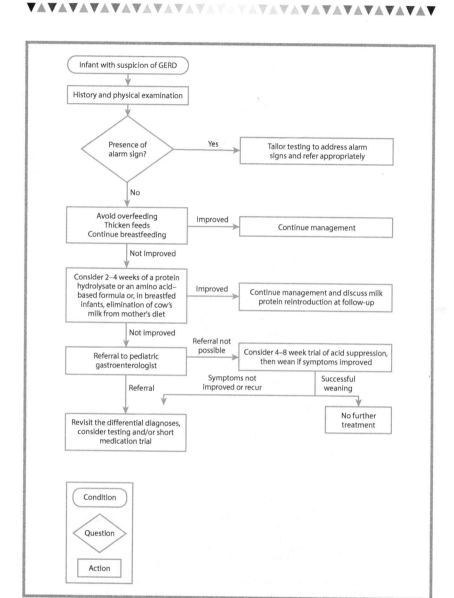

Figure 8-1. Evaluation and Management of an Infant With Symptoms Suggestive of Gastroesophageal Reflux Disease

Abbreviation: GERD, gastroesophageal reflux disease.

Adapted with permission from Rosen R, Vandenplas Y, Singendonk M, et al. Pediatric gastroesophageal reflux clinical practice guidelines: joint recommendations of the North American Society for Pediatric Gastroenterology, Hepatology, and Nutrition and the European Society for Pediatric Gastroenterology, Hepatology, and Nutrition. *J Pediatr Gastroenterol Nutr.* 2018;66(3):516–554.

▼▲▼▲▼▲▼▲▼▲▼▲▼▲▼▲▼   ▼▲▼▲▼▲▼▲▼▲▼▲▼▲▼▲▼

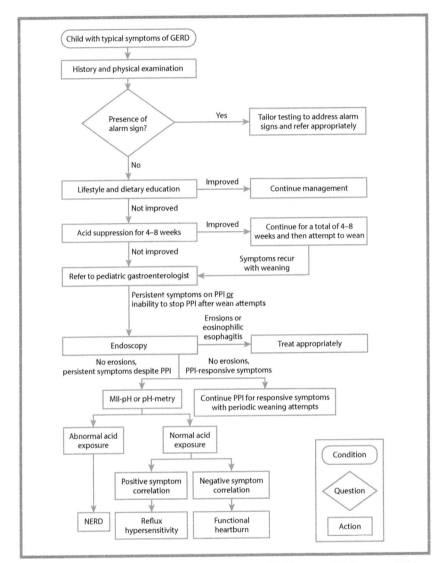

Figure 8-2. Evaluation and Management of a Child or an Adolescent With Symptoms Suggestive of Gastroesophageal Reflux Disease

Abbreviations: GERD, gastroesophageal reflux disease; MII-pH, multichannel intraluminal impedance-pH; NERD, nonerosive reflux disease; PPI, proton pump inhibitors.

Adapted with permission from Rosen R, Vandenplas Y, Singendonk M, et al. Pediatric gastroesophageal reflux clinical practice guidelines: joint recommendations of the North American Society for Pediatric Gastroenterology, Hepatology, and Nutrition and the European Society for Pediatric Gastroenterology, Hepatology, and Nutrition. *J Pediatr Gastroenterol Nutr.* 2018;66(3):516–554.

disease (Evidence Level III). Endoscopy may not be able to detect mild narrowing of the esophagus or achalasia, and it cannot be used to evaluate motility disorders or intestinal malrotation.

Barium Contrast Study

Indications for an upper GI barium contrast study in GERD include ruling out anatomic abnormalities that cause symptoms similar to those of GERD, such as esophageal stricture, achalasia, gastric outlet obstruction, antral or duodenal web, and intestinal malrotation (Evidence Level III). An upper GI barium contrast study also can be useful in evaluating children with a history of antireflux surgery who continue to have persistent reflux symptoms; the procedure can help differentiate an obstructing fundoplication from a slipped or loose fundoplication. An upper GI study is less useful in diagnosing GERD (Evidence Level III). Observation of GER during a contrast study does not enable the clinician to differentiate between physiological GER and GERD. Performing an upper GI barium contrast study in infants and children with uncomplicated GERD is not supported by the literature or by clinical practice.

Gastric Scintigraphy

Gastric scintigraphy records the movement of food or formula labeled with technetium Tc 99m and is the standard method for measuring gastric emptying. Gastroparesis, or delayed gastric emptying without mechanical obstruction, might contribute to GERD and can be detected via gastric scintigraphy. This study also can detect postprandial reflux and aspiration, but it can miss late postprandial reflux events and is neither sensitive nor specific for the diagnosis of GERD.

Manometry or Motility Studies

Manometry and other upper GI tract motility studies help distinguish between normal GI physiology and neuromuscular diseases. High-resolution esophageal manometry can clarify the role of transient lower esophageal sphincter relaxation in patients with GERD and detect abnormalities of peristalsis, bolus transit, and esophageal outlet obstruction. However, neither manometry nor motility testing has a role in the diagnosis of GERD in infants and children in whom there are no concerns regarding an underlying neuromuscular disease.

▼▲▼▲▼▲▼▲▼▲▼▲▼▲ ▲▼▲▼▲▼▲▼▲▼▲▼▲▼

MANAGEMENT

Lifestyle Modifications for Infants

For the infant with regurgitation that does not cause distress, parental education and adjustment of the feeding regimen may be enough to control symptoms. Uncomplicated regurgitation generally resolves by age 12 to 18 months. Avoiding overfeeding can help decrease vomiting (Evidence Level III). The addition of thickening agents such as rice cereal has also been shown to decrease vomiting but does not decrease the reflux index or frequency of acidic reflux events (Evidence Level II-A).

Prone positioning has been shown to decrease acidic reflux events when compared with supine positioning. However, the risk of mortality from sudden infant death syndrome far outweighs the risk of mortality from GERD; thus, supine positioning during sleep is recommended. Lying supine with the head of the bed elevated has not been shown to be more effective than lying flat.

Given the overlap in clinical presentation between GERD and cow's milk protein allergy, a 2-week trial of a protein hydrolysate or an amino acid–based formula may help differentiate the 2 processes. Current practice guidelines recommend a trial of an extensively hydrolyzed formula or amino acid–based formula in patients who have not responded to more conservative therapies before undergoing a trial of acid suppression. If the infant is breastfed, the mother should try a milk-free diet. A trial of at least 2 weeks is needed to allow mucosal healing, as symptomatic improvement typically is not immediate.

Lifestyle Modifications for Children and Adolescents

Children and adolescents should avoid caffeine, chocolate, alcohol, and spicy foods if these foods trigger symptoms. Chocolate, alcohol, and high-fat foods can reduce lower esophageal sphincter (LES) pressure and may lead to increased reflux. Weight loss in an obese patient may also improve symptoms, as obesity is associated with GERD.

Empiric Trial of Acid Suppression

A trial of acid suppression can be used for treatment and to aid in making a diagnosis of GERD (Evidence Level III). However, the evidence to support its use in infants and younger children is limited. Current practice guidelines recommend limiting acid suppression by conducting empiric trials of 4 to 8 weeks for GERD symptoms. **Table 8-3** provides dosing guidelines for the most common medications used in the treatment of GERD.

Table 8-3. Dosing Guidelines for Medications Commonly Used in Treatment of Children With Gastroesophageal Reflux Disease

Drugs	Recommended pediatric dosages	Maximum dosages[a] (mg)
Histamine-2 Receptor Antagonists		
Ranitidine	5–10 mg/kg/d	300
Cimetidine	30–40 mg/kg/d	800
Nizatidine	10–20 mg/kg/d	300
Famotidine	1 mg/kg/d	40
Proton Pump Inhibitors		
Omeprazole	1–4 mg/kg/d	40
Lansoprazole	2 mg/kg/d for infants	30
Esomeprazole	10 mg/d (weight <20 kg) or 20 mg/d (weight >20 kg)	40
Pantoprazole	1–2 mg/kg/d	40
Prokinetics		
Metoclopramide	0.4–0.9 mg/kg/d	60
Domperidone	0.8–0.9 mg/kg/d	30
Baclofen	0.5 mg/kg/d	80
Antacids and Protective Agents		
Mg alginate plus simethicone	2.5 mL tid (weight <5 kg) or 5 mL tid (weight >5 kg)	NA
Sodium alginate	225 mg sodium alginate and 87.5 mg magnesium alginate in a total 0.65 g 1 sachet/d (weight <4.54 kg) or 2 sachets/d (weight >4.54 kg)	NA
Sucralfate	40–80 mg/kg/d divided into 4 doses/d	4,000

Abbreviations: Mg, magnesium; NA, no data available; tid, 3 times per day.

[a] Maximum dosages are based on adult dosage; expressed per day.

Adapted with permission from Rosen R, Vandenplas Y, Singendonk M, et al. Pediatric gastroesophageal reflux clinical practice guidelines: joint recommendations of the North American Society for Pediatric Gastroenterology, Hepatology, and Nutrition and the European Society for Pediatric Gastroenterology, Hepatology, and Nutrition. *J Pediatr Gastroenterol Nutr.* 2018;66(3):516–554.

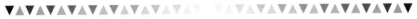

Histamine-2 Receptor Antagonists

Histamine-2 receptor antagonists (H2RAs) decrease acidic reflux events and improve healing of the esophageal mucosa compared with placebo (Evidence Level I). The H2RAs generally are well tolerated in children and are considered first-line treatment for infants. However, H2RAs are usually less effective than proton pump inhibitors (PPIs). Adverse effects include irritability, headache, somnolence, diarrhea, and constipation.

Proton Pump Inhibitors

Proton pump inhibitors are superior to H2RAs for treatment of symptoms and mucosal healing in adults, although the evidence is less clear in children (Evidence Level 1). PPIs also can increase gastric emptying, and, unlike H2RAs, tend to maintain their effect with long-term use. However, up to 14% of children treated with PPIs experience adverse effects, most commonly headache, diarrhea, constipation, and nausea. The risk of community-acquired pneumonia and gastroenteritis also may be increased with the use of PPIs. Further, use of PPIs in infants is controversial, as studies have not shown a reduction in symptoms when compared with placebo. In addition, PPI use may increase the risk of necrotizing enterocolitis in infants.

Prokinetic Agents

Prokinetic agents increase gastric emptying and may decrease reflux events by decompressing the stomach. Prokinetic agents are not recommended for routine GERD treatment, particularly given the side effect profiles of many of these medications, but they can be considered in patients with documented delayed gastric emptying (Evidence Level III).

Antacids and Surface Protective Agents

Older children and adolescents can take antacids after meals to quickly treat GERD symptoms. Evidence for their use in younger children is limited, and the long-term use of antacids is not recommended given the risk of increased plasma aluminum levels with aluminum-containing antacids and milk-alkali syndrome with calcium carbonate–containing antacids. Antacids are not recommended as a single-agent treatment for GERD in children.

Sucralfate is a surface protective agent that acts by coating gastric erosions when exposed to an acidic environment, thereby potentially encouraging healing of esophagitis. However, given the limited amount of information available about the safety of sucralfate in children, it is not recommended as single-agent therapy for GERD, and treatment is typically limited to fewer than 10 days.

Antireflux Surgery

Fundoplication can eliminate GER, including physiological GER, but it is reserved for children in whom optimal medical therapy has failed, as well as for children who depend on long-term medical therapy or who have developed life-threatening complications of GERD. Evidence in children regarding complications and long-term outcomes remains limited.

LONG-TERM CONSIDERATIONS

Although GER and GERD are common in infants, children, and adolescents, the diagnosis and management of these disorders can be challenging. A thorough clinical history is critical to identify signs that might suggest an underlying etiology other than GER or GERD. Diagnostic testing is typically not needed for a child with uncomplicated GER or GERD. Management differs based on age and clinical presentation, and it can involve lifestyle changes, dietary modification, and acid suppression. Antireflux surgery is reserved for children with refractory GERD, often when associated with life-threatening complications. Recent clinical guidelines provide a framework for the evaluation and management of children with GER and GERD (Evidence Level III).

SUGGESTED READING

Baird DC, Harker DJ, Karmes AS. Diagnosis and treatment of gastroesophageal reflux in infants and children. *Am Fam Physician.* 2015;92(8):705–714

Horvath A, Dziechciarz P, Szajewska H. The effect of thickened-feed interventions on gastro-esophageal reflux in infants: systematic review and meta-analysis of randomized, controlled trials. *Pediatrics.* 2008;122(6):e1268–e1277

Khan M, Santana J, Donnellan C, Preston C, Moayyedi P. Medical treatments in the short term management of reflux oesophagitis. *Cochrane Database Syst Rev.* 2007;(2):CD003244

Nelson SP, Chen EH, Syniar GM, Christoffel KK. Prevalence of symptoms of gastroesophageal reflux during childhood: a pediatric practice-based survey. Pediatric Practice Research Group. *Arch Pediatr Adolesc Med.* 2000;154(2):150–154

Rosen R, Vandenplas Y, Singendonk M, et al. Pediatric gastroesophageal reflux clinical practice guidelines: joint recommendations of the North American Society for Pediatric Gastroenterology, Hepatology, and Nutrition and the European Society for Pediatric Gastroenterology, Hepatology, and Nutrition. *J Pediatr Gastroenterol Nutr.* 2018;66(3):516–554

Sullivan JS, Sundaram SS. Gastroesophageal reflux. *Pediatr Rev.* 2012;33(6):243–254

van der Pol RJ, Smits MJ, van Wijk MP, Omari TI, Tabbers MM, Benninga MA. Efficacy of proton-pump inhibitors in children with gastroesophageal reflux disease: a systematic review. *Pediatrics.* 2011;127(5):925–935

Vandenplas Y, Rudolph CD, Di Lorenzo C, et al; North American Society for Pediatric Gastroenterology, Hepatology, and Nutrition; European Society for Pediatric Gastroenterology, Hepatology, and Nutrition. Pediatric gastroesophageal reflux clinical practice guidelines: joint recommendations of the North American Society for Pediatric Gastroenterology, Hepatology, and Nutrition (NASPGHAN) and the European Society for Pediatric Gastroenterology, Hepatology, and Nutrition (ESPGHAN). *J Pediatr Gastroenterol Nutr.* 2009;49(4):498–547

Gastrointestinal Bleeding

Lay Har Cheng, MD, MSPH, and Victor M. Piñeiro, MD

OVERVIEW

Gastrointestinal (GI) bleeding is an anxiety-producing experience for parents and children. Fortunately, most common causes of GI bleeding are minor and self-limited. However, though most children with GI bleeding are clinically stable, in rare cases, GI bleeding can be massive and life threatening. A rapid assessment of the child's hemodynamic status is important, and, if necessary, hemodynamic stabilization should take priority over further diagnostic evaluation. For a child with hemodynamic instability and ongoing GI bleeding, early gastroenterology and surgical consultations are imperative for possible emergency endoscopic or surgical therapy (Evidence Level III).

In the stable patient, a detailed history and physical examination are necessary to help discern whether the source of the bleeding is gastrointestinal, as well as to identify children at greatest risk of GI bleeding. Upper gastrointestinal (UGI) bleeding, defined as bleeding proximal to the ligament of Treitz, may present as vomiting of gross blood (hematemesis) or coffee-ground vomiting caused by degradation of the heme by gastric acid. Massive UGI bleeding can present with melena (black tarry stools), with or without hematemesis, or with hematochezia (red bloody stools) in the setting of rapid transit due to the cathartic effects of blood. Lower gastrointestinal (LGI) bleeding, or bleeding distal to the ligament of Treitz, may present with bright red blood on the toilet tissue after passing a bowel movement, small clots of blood mixed with the stool, bloody diarrhea, or hematochezia. The clinical presentation for occult GI bleeding may be unexplained fatigue, pallor, or iron deficiency anemia.

CAUSES

The primary causes of GI bleeding vary by age of the patient, clinical presentation, associated symptoms, and clinical appearance of the child. Upper gastrointestinal bleeding may present as small-volume bright blood or coffee-ground emesis in a child who appears well or as a massive hematemesis or melena (**Table 9-1**). Occasionally, a child is initially asymptomatic, only to develop signs and symptoms of cardiovascular collapse with ongoing severe GI bleeding. As in UGI bleeding, the primary causes of LGI bleeding also vary by age of the patient, associated symptoms, and the child's appearance (**Table 9-2**). Melena often is caused by a UGI source (see **Table 9-1**).

Table 9-1. Main Causes of Upper Gastrointestinal Bleeding,[a] by Age and Patient's Appearance

Age	Well-Appearing Child	Ill-Appearing Child
Newborn/ infant	Swallowed maternal blood Vitamin K deficiency Reflux esophagitis Reactive gastritis Milk-protein sensitivity Vomiting-induced hematemesis (prolapse gastropathy syndrome) Gastrointestinal duplications	Stress gastritis or ulcer Coagulopathy (DIC) Mallory-Weiss tear Duodenal/gastric web Bowel obstruction
Preschool (2–5 y)	Vomiting-induced hematemesis (prolapse gastropathy syndrome) Acid-peptic disease Mallory-Weiss tear	Esophageal varices (liver disease) Hemorrhagic gastritis Stress gastritis or ulcer Caustic ingestion Bowel obstruction
Older child/ adolescent	Vomiting-induced hematemesis (prolapse gastropathy syndrome) Mallory-Weiss tear Reflux esophagitis Reactive gastritis	Esophageal varices (liver disease) Hemorrhagic gastritis Stress gastritis or ulcer Bowel obstruction Dieulafoy lesion

Abbreviation: DIC, disseminated intravascular coagulation.

[a] Rare causes of upper gastrointestinal bleeding: vascular malformation, hemobilia, intestinal duplication, vasculitis, aortoenteric fistulae.

▼▲▼▲▼▲▼▲▼▲▼▲▼▲▼ ▼▲▼▲▼▲▼▲▼▲▼▲▼▲▼

Table 9-2. Main Causes of Lower Gastrointestinal Bleeding,[a] by Age and Patient's Appearance

Age	Well-Appearing Child	Ill-Appearing Child
Newborn/ infant	Allergic proctocolitis Anal fissure Nodular lymphoid hyperplasia Intestinal duplication Infectious colitis Hemorrhagic disease of the newborn Meckel diverticulum	Necrotizing enterocolitis Malrotation with volvulus Infectious colitis Hirschsprung disease enterocolitis Intussusception
Preschool (2–5 y)	Anal fissure Juvenile polyp Perianal streptococcal cellulitis Rectal prolapse Meckel diverticulum Nodular lymphoid hyperplasia Inflammatory bowel disease	Infectious colitis Intussusception malrotation with volvulus Henoch-Schönlein purpura Hemolytic uremic syndrome Ulcerative colitis
Older child/ adolescent	Anal fissure Infectious colitis Hemorrhoid Polyp Inflammatory bowel disease Meckel diverticulum	Infectious colitis Ulcerative colitis Henoch-Schönlein purpura

[a] Rare causes of bleeding: vascular malformation, hemobilia, intestinal duplication, intestinal ischemia.

INITIAL PRESENTATION AND ASSESSMENT

Based on the patient's answers to specific questions, the physician can approx-imate the severity, source, and duration of bleeding and determine where the patient needs to be sent (Evidence Level III) (**Box 9-1**). Large-volume bleeding or an ill appearance would prompt emergent transport to a local emergency department. A social and family history may direct the physician to specific conditions that could be evident for the first time. In addition, various foods and

Box 9-1. Historical Information (Open-Ended Questions)

- Describe the location, quantity, and appearance of the bleeding.
- What are the physical appearance and vital signs of the patient (if available)?
- What medical conditions does the child have (eg, liver disease, inflammatory bowel disease)?
- What medication is the child receiving (eg, anticoagulants, nonsteroidal anti-inflammatory drugs)?

History
- Description of onset, location, duration, occurrence
- Exposure to raw food, reptiles, travel, or toxins
- Foreign body ingestion
- Exposure to others with similar symptoms
- Ingestion of specific foods or medications
- Other associated symptoms (ie, mouth sores, pain, rashes, vomiting, swelling, headaches, neck pain, chest pain, diarrhea, fevers, bruising, and infections)
- Medications (ie, nonsteroidal anti-inflammatory drugs, warfarin, hepatotoxins, antibiotics)

Review of systems
- Gastrointestinal disorders
- Liver disease
- Bleeding diatheses
- Anesthesia reactions

Family history
- Gastrointestinal disorders (eg, polyps, ulcers, colitis)
- Liver disease
- Bleeding diatheses
- Anesthesia reactions

Reproduced with permission from Wyllie R, Hyams JS, Kay M, eds. *Pediatric Gastrointestinal and Liver Disease*. 5th ed. Philadelphia, PA: Elsevier; 2016:145.

▼▲▼▲▼▲▼▲▼▲▼▲▼▲▼   ▼ ▲▼▲▼▲▼▲▼▲▼▲▼▲▼

medications can cause stools or emesis to falsely appear to contain blood (eg, candies, fruit juices, beets, blueberries, iron, bismuth).

UPPER GASTROINTESTINAL BLEEDING

Initial Evaluation

The clinician can best confirm the presence of blood in gastric contents via the gastric occult blood test, if a specimen can be obtained. Epistaxis, oropharyngeal bleeding, and hemoptysis should be considered and ruled out in cases of suspected UGI bleeding. For newborns or breastfeeding infants, swallowed maternal blood must be considered, and the Apt-Downey test can be used to distinguish fetal hemoglobin from adult hemoglobin. The initial evaluation of children with UGI bleeding should include a targeted physical examination (**Box 9-2**) and laboratory evaluation (**Box 9-3**).

The evaluation requires a careful individualized approach based on associated symptoms, signs, and severity of bleeding. Initial hemoglobin and hematocrit tests are critical but may underestimate the degree of bleeding. A normal saline gastric lavage can be used to confirm the presence of esophageal

Box 9-2. Focused Physical Examination

Vital signs: HR, BP (orthostasis), pulse pressure, urine output

General: appearance (well or ill), fever, mental status

Head, eyes, ears, nose, and throat: trauma, petechiae, lip and buccal pigmentation, epistaxis, erythema or burns to posterior pharynx

Cardiovascular: tachycardia, heart murmur, capillary refill

Abdomen: tenderness, splenomegaly, hepatomegaly, ascites

Rectal: gross blood, melena, skin tags, tenderness, fissure, fistula, hemorrhoids, fecal occult blood

Abbreviations: BP, blood pressure; HR, heart rate.

Box 9-3. Laboratory Evaluation

- Complete blood cell count
- Prothrombin time/international normalized ratio
- Complete metabolic profile
- Type and screen
- If significant loss: type and cross, fibrinogen level
- Stool studies (if indicated by history): stool culture, *Escherichia coli* O157:H7, *Shigella, Salmonella, Yersinia, Campylobacter*; *Clostridium difficile* toxin; *Cryptosporidium* and *Giardia* antigen assay
- Erythrocyte sedimentation rate, C-reactive protein
- Hemoccult and Gastroccult testing

or gastric bleeding, as well as to identify active bleeding (Evidence Level III). Note that duodenal bleeding may be missed on gastric lavage because the duodenum is transpyloric. Upper gastrointestinal bleeding usually is self-limited in children. However, patients with ongoing bleeding warrant urgent evaluation (see **Box 9-3**).

Additional Evaluation

Radiographic and endoscopic studies may be useful in evaluating a child with UGI bleeding (**Table 9-3**). Esophagogastroduodenoscopy (EGD) is the preferred method to confirm the diagnosis and possibly treat the bleeding lesion (Evidence Level III; see Therapy section); however, necessity and timing of EGD depend on clinical presentation and suspected source. If the patient has hematemesis or a positive finding on nasogastric lavage, radiographic testing is rarely indicated unless the EGD results are negative. However, radiographic studies may be helpful in certain clinical scenarios. Plain chest and abdominal radiographs can be used to identify a foreign body, an esophageal or a bowel perforation, or a bowel obstruction. Abdominal ultrasonography can identify portal hypertension responsible for esophageal or gastric varices. In the setting of brisk bleeding (ie, ≥0.5 mL/min), angiography allows for identification of

▼▲▼▲▼▲▼▲▼▲▼▲▼▲▼▲ ▼ ▼ ▲▼▲▼▲▼▲▼▲▼▲▼▲▼▲▼

Table 9-3. Imaging Studies and Associated Indications

Test	Indication
Chest and abdominal radiographs	Foreign body obstruction, vomiting
Upper gastrointestinal series	Dysphagia, odynophagia, drooling, obstruction, vomiting
Barium enema	Suspected stricture, intussusception, Hirschsprung disease
Ultrasound (Doppler recommended for liver disease)	Portal hypertension, intussusception
Meckel scan	Meckel diverticulum
Tagged RBC scan	Obscure gastrointestinal bleeding
MRI/CT	Obstruction Suspected inflammatory bowel disease Obscure gastrointestinal bleeding
Angiography	Suspected arteriovenous malformation

Abbreviations: CT, computed tomography; MRI, magnetic resonance imaging; RBC, red blood cell count.

the bleed, as well as for therapy by means of embolization through placement of coils.

Therapy

Fluid resuscitation with prompt intravascular volume replacement is the highest priority for both UGI and LGI bleeding (Evidence Level II). Treatment options for UGI bleeding include acid reduction, vasoconstriction, and cytoprotection (**Box 9-4**). Antacids, H2-receptor antagonists, and proton pump inhibitors (PPIs) can aid in treating suspected acid-peptic disease, as well as in reducing acid injury to an existing mucosal defect. Although the current guidelines recommend high-dose intravenous PPI bolus followed by a continuous infusion, intermittent PPI therapy has been found to be safe and effective for patients with significant UGI bleeding who are awaiting an upper endoscopy (Evidence Level III; adults, Evidence Level I). Octreotide can be used to reduce splanchnic blood flow, particularly in the setting of portal hypertension.

Box 9-4. Treatment of Gastrointestinal Bleeding

Supportive care
- Intravenous fluids (isotonic saline or Ringer lactate)
- Blood products (packed red blood cells, fresh-frozen plasma, platelets)
- Pressors (eg, norepinephrine, dopamine)

Specific care
- Proton pump inhibitors (eg, intravenous pantoprazole)
- Somatostatin analogue (octreotide)
- Cytoprotective agent (eg, sucralfate, aluminum-containing antacids)

Endoscopic therapy
- Injection (sclerosant, epinephrine, normal saline, hypertonic saline)
- Coagulation (bipolar, monopolar, heater probe, laser, argon plasma)
- Hemostatic powder
- Variceal injection and ligation
- Band ligation
- Polypectomy
- Endoscopic clip or loop

Interventional radiology
- Angiography (eg, placement of gelatin sponge, microcoil embalization, cyanoacrylate)

Sucralfate is activated in an acidic environment (pH <4) to form a buffer and an insoluble barrier that binds to proteins on the surface of ulcers. However, sucralfate should be avoided in patients with chronic renal failure because of its aluminum content.

▼▲▼▲▼▲▼▲▼▲▼▲▼▲▼ ▼▲▼▲▼▲▼▲▼▲▼▲▼▲▼

Endoscopic therapy includes electrocoagulation, laser photocoagulation, argon plasma coagulation, injection of epinephrine and sclerosants, band ligation, placement of endoscopic clips or loops, and use of hemostatic powder. These modalities carry the risk of intestinal necrosis, perforation, and obstruction, but their use can be critical to stop ongoing bleeding.

The clinician should pursue a surgical consultation before performing any endoscopic intervention in which the risk of severe bleeding is high. Surgical intervention should be reserved for patients in whom hemodynamic stability is tenuous or bleeding is uncontrolled. An exploratory laparotomy may be necessary in children with a GI perforation or an obstruction.

LOWER GASTROINTESTINAL BLEEDING

History and Physical Examination

A detailed history and physical examination can help the clinician narrow the list of potential causes of LGI bleeding. A family history of a first-degree relative with allergy, inflammatory bowel disease, familial adenomatous polyposis, hereditary hemorrhagic telangiectasia, Ehlers-Danlos syndrome, or a bleeding disorder raises the possibility of the same disorder in the patient. A personal history of neonatal sepsis, omphalitis, umbilical catheterization, abdominal surgery, previous GI bleeding, hematologic abnormalities, or liver disease can further direct the clinician toward the most likely source of the LGI bleeding. Risk factors such as day care attendance and recent use of antibiotics raise the possibility of a bacterial or viral GI infection.

The clinical characteristics can also elucidate the most likely causes of the LGI bleeding (**tables 9-4** and **9-5**).

Initial Evaluation

Fecal occult blood testing (guaiac test) can confirm the presence of blood in the stool. Rarely, false-positive findings can occur from consumption of myoglobin or hemoglobin in meat or ascorbic acid in uncooked fruits and vegetables. Epistaxis, oropharyngeal bleeding, hemoptysis, hematuria, and menses should be considered and ruled out in cases of suspected LGI bleeding. For newborns or breastfeeding infants, swallowed maternal blood must be considered, and the Apt-Downey test can distinguish the presence of fetal hemoglobin from adult hemoglobin. In addition, the clinician must consider UGI bleeding, as it may present with melena, hematochezia, and anemia.

▼▲▼▲▼▲▼▲▼▲▼▲▼▲▼▲▼   ▼▲▼▲▼▲▼▲▼▲▼▲▼▲▼▲▼

Table 9-4. Principal Associated Gastrointestinal (GI) Symptoms in Relation to Underlying Cause(s) of Lower GI Bleeding

Amount of Blood Loss	Appearance of Blood	Characteristics of Stools	Pain	Underlying Disease
Small	Red	Hard	Yes (anorectal)	Anal fissure
Small to moderate	Red	Loose	Variable (abdominal)	Allergic proctocolitis, infectious colitis, hemolytic uremic syndrome, inflammatory bowel disease
Small to moderate	Red	Normal, coated with blood	No	Polyp
Moderate	Red to tarry	Normal	Yes (abdominal)	Henoch-Schönlein purpura
Moderate	Red to tarry, currant jelly	Normal	Yes (abdominal)	Intussusception
Moderate	Red to tarry	Loose	Yes (abdominal)	Hirschsprung disease enterocolitis
Large	Red to tarry	Normal	No	Meckel diverticulum, angiodysplasia

Reproduced with permission from Turck D, Michaud L. Lower gastrointestinal bleeding. In: Walker WA, Goulet OJ, Kleinman RE, Sherman PM, Shneider BL, Sanderson IR, eds. *Pediatric Gastrointestinal Disease: Pathophysiology, Diagnosis, Management*. 4th ed. Raleigh, NC: PMPH USA; 2004:268.

Table 9-5. Principal Physical Findings in Relation to the Underlying Cause(s) of Lower Gastrointestinal Bleeding

Location	Physical Finding	Underlying Disease
Abdomen	Hepatosplenomegaly, ascites, dilated venous channels on the abdomen, caput medusa	Portal hypertension
	Abdominal mass	Intussusception, IBD, intestinal duplication
Perineal area	Anal fissure	Constipation, Crohn disease
	Skin tag, fistula, abscess	Crohn disease, chronic granulomatous disease, immunodeficiency syndromes
	Hemorrhoids, rectal varicosities	Portal hypertension, constipation (adolescent)
	Rectal mass at digital rectal examination	Polyp
Skin and mucous membranes	Eczema	Food allergy
	Purpura	Henoch-Schönlein purpura, hemorrhagic disease, hemolytic uremic syndrome
	Jaundice, palmar erythema, spider angioma	Liver cirrhosis
	Digital clubbing	Liver cirrhosis, IBD
	Pyoderma gangrenosum	Ulcerative colitis
	Erythema nodosum	Crohn disease
	Telangiectasia	Hereditary hemorrhagic telangiectasia
	Soft tissue tumor (skull, mandible)	Gardner syndrome

▼▲▼▲▼▲▼▲▼▲▼▲▼▲▼▲▼ ▲▼▲▼▲▼▲▼▲▼▲▼▲▼▲▼

Table 9-5. Principal Physical Findings in Relation to the Underlying Cause(s) of Lower Gastrointestinal Bleeding (*continued*)

Location	Physical Finding	Underlying Disease
Skin and mucous membranes (*continued*)	Café au lait spots	Turcot syndrome
	Pigmentation of the lips, buccal mucosa, face	Peutz-Jeghers syndrome
	Alopecia, onychodystrophy, hyperpigmentation	Cronkhite-Canada syndrome
	Breast hypertrophy	Cowden disease
	Bluish soft nodules	Blue rubber bleb nevus syndrome
	Soft-tissue hypertrophy	Klippel-Trénaunay syndrome
Eye	Iritis	IBD
Joint	Arthritis	Henoch-Schönlein purpura, IBD
Growth	Failure to thrive	IBD, Hirschsprung disease
	Very short stature, webbed neck, widespread nipples	Turner syndrome

Abbreviation: IBD, inflammatory bowel disease.
Reproduced with permission from Turck D, Michaud L. Lower gastrointestinal bleeding. In: Walker WA, Goulet OJ, Kleinman RE, Sherman PM, Shneider BL, Sanderson IR, eds. *Pediatric Gastrointestinal Disease: Pathophysiology, Diagnosis, Management.* 4th ed. Raleigh, NC: PMPH USA; 2004:269.

The initial evaluation of children with LGI bleeding should include a targeted physical examination (see **Box 9-2**) and laboratory testing (see **Box 9-3**). A normal saline gastric lavage is useful to confirm UGI bleeding in the presence of large-volume melena or hematochezia (Evidence Level III).

▼△▼△▼△▼△▼△▼△▼△▼△ △ ▼△▼△▼△▼△▼△▼△▼△▼

Additional Evaluation

Radiographic studies are often performed and are especially helpful when trying to exclude a surgical emergency (see **Table 9-3**). Plain upright and supine abdominal radiographs should be obtained in patients suspected of having an obstruction, ischemia, or perforation. Barium enema should be avoided as part of an initial evaluation, as it will lead to delays in endoscopic and scintigraphic evaluation. Abdominal ultrasonography can be used to evaluate an abdominal mass or suspected intussusception. If findings are suspicious for intussusception, an air contrast enema is the next step for diagnostic confirmation and treatment. A colonoscopy is the procedure of choice for evaluating LGI bleeding. Small-bowel enteroscopy, available at certain centers only, allows for visualization, sampling, and endoscopic treatment of the small bowel between the ligament of Treitz and the ileocecal valve. Video capsule endoscopy can be used to evaluate the small bowel for bleeding and ulceration; however, it should be avoided in those with a potential partial obstruction that may prevent safe and effective passage of the camera.

Abdominal scintigraphy with technetium Tc 99m pertechnetate, also known as a Meckel scan, can be used to identify the heterotopic gastric mucosa in a Meckel diverticulum or an intestinal duplication. A radioisotope-tagged red blood cell bleeding scan performed with a sample of the patient's own red blood cells tagged with Tc 99m can identify sources of bleeding when the rate of blood loss is at least 0.05 to 0.2 mL/minute. Computed tomographic angiography has recently replaced the bleeding scan as the initial assessment tool because it may provide faster diagnosis and delineate vascular abnormalities; its sensitivity is similar to that of the bleeding scan. Angiography, which is helpful when the bleeding rate exceeds 0.5 mL/minute, has the added benefit of allowing for intraprocedure embolization or local infusion of vasopressin; however, it carries with it the risk of serious complications, including arterial spasm, arterial thrombosis, contrast reaction, and acute renal failure.

Therapy

Many of the medical or surgical treatment options for LGI bleeding are similar to those for UGI bleeding (see **Box 9-4**). Once colonic preparation (ie, cleanout) is complete, a colonoscopy can often identify the bleeding lesion. Other specific medical and surgical treatment options are tailored to the underlying cause of the bleeding, which is beyond the scope of this chapter.

SUGGESTED READING

Boyle JT. Gastrointestinal bleeding in infants and children. *Pediatr Rev.* 2008;29(2):39–52

Pai AK, Fox VL. Gastrointestinal bleeding and management. *Pediatr Clin North Am.* 2017;64(3):543–561

Kleinman RE, Goulet O-J, Mieli-Vergani G, Sanderson IR, Sherman PM, Shneider BL, eds. *Walker's Pediatric Gastrointestinal Disease: Physiology, Diagnosis, Management.* 6th ed. Raleigh, NC: PMPH USA; 2018

Wyllie R, Hyams JS, Kay M, eds. *Pediatric Gastrointestinal and Liver Disease.* 5th ed. Philadelphia, PA: Elsevier; 2016

Hepatitis, Viral

Vani V. Gopalareddy, MD

OVERVIEW

The hepatotropic viruses (hepatitis A through E) typically cause predominant hepatic injury and dysfunction unlike those in other viral illnesses that lead to hepatic inflammation as part of a more widespread systemic disease process. Most viruses that cause hepatitis can be confirmed by a specific antibody or by nuclear antigen detection. Viral hepatitis may present as acute, chronic, or fulminant with acute liver failure.

About 10% of cases of severe hepatitis are caused by other viral illnesses, such as Epstein-Barr virus, cytomegalovirus, herpes simplex virus, adenovirus, parvovirus B19, human herpesvirus-6, enteroviruses such as coxsackie, and echoviruses.

HEPATITIS A VIRUS

Hepatitis A virus (HAV) is the most common form of acute viral hepatitis in the world. Children younger than 10 years usually have an asymptomatic infection; the likelihood of a symptomatic infection increases with age. Hepatitis A virus is self-limiting and does not lead to chronic hepatitis. Risk factors for transmission include household exposure, day care attendance, and travel to endemic areas. Hepatis A virus is spread through fecal-oral transmission, and patients with HAV are most infectious during the prodromal phase; however, HAV may be detected in stool for longer periods in neonates and young children.

Differential Diagnosis

Box 10-1 lists the variety of causes of acute and chronic hepatitis in children. Signs and symptoms of secondary disorders, a history of travel, and pathogen exposure, as well as results of diagnostic tests provide important information regarding the most likely etiology. Preliminary liver screening tests include liver enzymes, synthetic function, and cholestatic parameters. Viral serologic testing

Box 10-1. Differential Diagnosis for Acute Infectious Hepatitis

Viral hepatitis (most common)
- Typical acute viral hepatitis
  —Hepatitis A, B, C, D, or E
  —Cytomegalovirus
  —Mononucleosis
  —Coxsackievirus
- Potentially severe hepatitis (especially in immunocompromised patients)
  —Herpes simplex virus
  —Varicella

Bacterial hepatitis
- Leptospirosis (associated with animal or tick-borne exposure)
- Q fever
- Rocky Mountain Spotted Fever
- Secondary syphilis
- Typhoid fever
- Overwhelming infection (sepsis)
- Liver abscess (especially in immunocompromised hosts or those with underlying cancer)
- Fitz-Hugh-Curtis syndrome (*Neisseria gonorrhoeae*)

Parasite
- *Entamoeba histolytica* (liver abscess)
- Toxocariasis
- Liver trematodes (liver flukes)

Fungal causes
- *Candida albicans* (liver abscess, especially in immunocompromised patients)

studies help identify the causative agent. Moreover, an abdominal ultrasound scan is essential to exclude obstruction and structural disorders. If the underlying hepatic disease remains obscure or parenchymal liver damage needs to be defined, a liver biopsy may be performed.

Clinical Features

The prodromal symptoms of hepatitis A usually develop after a 2- to 6-week incubation period. They are nonspecific and include anorexia, nausea, vomiting, tiredness, and fever. Children may develop a gastroenteritis-like illness with a predominance of vomiting and diarrhea. Jaundice, tender hepatomegaly, and dark urine have also been reported in some cases of hepatitis A. Splenomegaly, posterior cervical lymphadenopathy, and arthritis may occur, but they are rare. Some children may have atypical symptoms such as prolonged cholestasis, ascites, relapsing hepatitis, or fulminant hepatitis. Most children experience an uncomplicated course, with complete recovery within 2 to 6 months of symptom onset. Jaundice usually resolves in 2 weeks. Some patients may have prolonged cholestasis. Extrahepatic complications, such as autoimmune hemolytic anemia, aplastic anemia, acute pancreatitis, and acalculous cholecystitis, as well as renal and neurological complications, can occur, but they are rare. Children with HAV should not attend school or child care settings for 1 week after the onset of symptoms. Hospitalization generally is not required.

Improved hygiene and sanitation are the most effective strategies for preventing viral hepatitis. Passive immunization and active immunizations are available, particularly for high-risk populations.

Evaluation

Nonspecific Tests

Elevated transaminases (aspartate aminotransferase [AST] and alanine aminotransferase [ALT]) and bilirubin (nonspecific) are almost invariably present in HAV. Bilirubin levels peak later and decrease more slowly than transaminases. Laboratory test results may be abnormal for 2 or more months. In HAV, an abdominal ultrasound examination typically reveals nonspecific findings such as hepatomegaly, thickened gallbladder wall, periportal echogenicity, and periportal lymphadenopathy.

Confirmatory/Serologic Test

In HAV, anti-HAV IgM antibodies peak during the acute illness and may persist for up to 4 to 6 months after infection. The anti-HAV IgG antibody appears early, peaks during the convalescent phase, and persists for the rest of the patient's life (immunity).

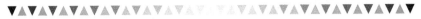

Management

No specific antiviral therapy is available for acute HAV infection. Management is mainly supportive care and includes rest, hydration, and analgesia. In general, prolonged cholestasis should be managed with antipruritic therapy and fat-soluble vitamin supplementation (Evidence Level III). Occasionally, steroids are used to minimize inflammation and provide quicker resolution of symptoms. Liver transplantation should be considered for cases complicated by acute liver failure.

CHRONIC VIRAL HEPATITIS (HBV AND HCV)

Chronic viral hepatitis caused by HBV and HCV is the leading cause of chronic liver disease worldwide. Acute infection is more common with HBV than HCV in childhood. Chronic asymptomatic hepatitis with HBV or HCV can lead to chronic liver disease. Late development of hepatocellular carcinoma (HCC) is a particular concern with both HBV and HCV.

Hepatitis B

Clinical Features

Hepatitis B may rarely present as an acute infection or as fulminant hepatitis, but such presentations are usually associated with hepatitis D virus coinfection. Infection typically is asymptomatic and leads to chronic sequelae, including carrier state in 10% to 95% of cases and chronic hepatitis in 5% to 10% of cases (but 90% if vertically acquired). After acute HBV infection, 90% of children recover spontaneously, but about 1% develop acute fulminant hepatitis. The chronic HBV infection may be completely asymptomatic or associated with mild elevations of transaminases. Children with chronic HBV infection have a 25% lifetime risk of developing cirrhosis or HCC.

Perinatal transmission remains the main source of infection in childhood. Vertical transmission is highest if the mother is HBeAg positive. The likelihood of developing chronic hepatitis is highest if the infection is acquired in infancy. Hepatitis B virus transmission can be effectively prevented by immunization, antenatal screening, and screening of blood products and organ donors. Hepatitis B vaccine should be administered to all infants at birth. Hepatitis B immunoglobulin is indicated for high-risk infants born to mothers who are HBV carriers. The vaccine is effective in more than 97% of newborns and lasts for 10 to 15 years. Tenofovir disoproxil fumarate (TDF) treatment started at 28 weeks of gestation in HBsAg-positive mothers with HBV viral load

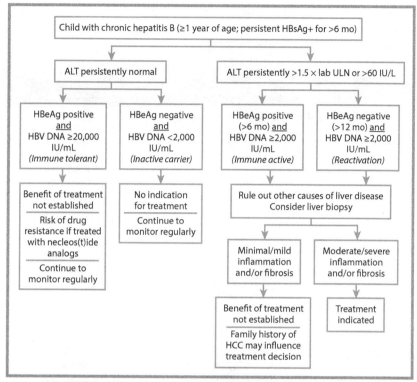

Figure 10-1. Algorithm for Monitoring and for Treatment Considerations in Children With Chronic Hepatitis B Virus Infection

Abbreviations: ALT, alanine aminotransferase; HBeAg, hepatitis Be antigen; HBsAg, hepatitis B surface antigen; HBV, hepatitis B virus; HCC, hepatocellular carcinoma; IU, international units; ULN, upper limit of normal.

Reproduced with permission from Jonas MM, Block JM, Haber BA, et al. Treatment of children with chronic hepatitis B virus infection in the United States: patient selection and therapeutic options. *Hepatology*. 2010;52(6):2192–2205.

greater than 200,000 IU/mL helps to prevent maternal to child transmission of hepatitis B.

Chronic HBV infection is the persistence of HBsAg for longer than 6 months. Most children with chronic HBV infection in the immune-tolerant phase are asymptomatic and do not require treatment. These children can develop progressive liver disease and complications in adulthood. Spontaneous HBeAg seroconversion rates vary during childhood and until late adolescence.

Chronic HBV infection is characterized by 4 immunologic phases of disease (**Table 10-1**). Most children remain in the immune-tolerant phase until late childhood and do not need treatment.

Table 10-1. Phases of Chronic Hepatitis B Virus Infection

Phase	Laboratory Results and Histology	Comments
Immune tolerant	• HBsAg and HBeAg detectable • HBV DNA >20,000 IU/mL (>1 million copies/mL) • ALT normal • Absent or minimal liver inflammation/ fibrosis	• Biopsy not indicated • Antiviral therapies generally ineffective
HBeAg+ immune active	• HBsAg and HBeAg remain detectable • HBV DNA >20,000 IU/mL (>1 million copies/mL) • ALT persistently elevated • Liver inflammation and fibrosis can develop	• Biopsy indicated • Consider treatment
Inactive HBsAg "carrier"	• HBsAg present • HBeAg negative, anti-HBe present • HBV DNA <2,000 IU/mL (<10,000 copies/ mL) or undetectable • ALT normal • Absent or minimal liver inflammation/ fibrosis	• Biopsy not indicated • Risk of HCC • Continued monitoring recommended
Reactivation or HBeAg-negative immune active	• HBsAg present • HBeAg negative, anti-HBe present • HBV DNA >2,000 IU/mL (>10,000 copies/ mL) • ALT level normal or elevated • Active liver inflammation with or without fibrosis	• Occurs in 20%– 30% of patients • Called "e-Ag negative" hepatitis B • Biopsy indicated • Treatment is long term

Abbreviations: ALT, alanine aminotransferase; HBeAg, hepatitis Be antigen; HBsAg, hepatitis B surface antigen; HBV, hepatitis B virus; HCC, hepatocellular carcinoma; IU, international units.

Reproduced with permission from Jonas MM, Block JM, Haber BA, et al. Treatment of children with chronic hepatitis B virus infection in the United States: patient selection and therapeutic options. *Hepatology*. 2010;52(6):2192–2205.

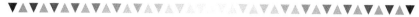

Evaluation

Serum HBsAg with anti-HBs is the most effective screening tool for HBV infection. Children found to be HBsAg positive should be retested 6 months later to document chronic infection. Baseline liver function tests are recommended (ALT, AST, bilirubin), as well as a complete blood cell count, HBV DNA load, HBeAg, alpha-fetoprotein, and a liver ultrasound examination.

Management

All children with chronic HBV infection should be monitored annually. Treatment is indicated for children in the immune-active phase with consistently (>6 months) abnormal ALT levels to reduce long-term complications. An observation period of 3 to 6 months before treatment is prudent to determine if spontaneous HBeAg seroconversion occurs. Interferon-based therapies are no longer used because of significant side effects and poor efficacy. Interferon clears viral infection in only 20% to 40% of patients. Typical first-line treatment options include oral nucleoside(tide) therapies. Only 23% of children experience seroconversion after lamivudine treatment, 26% of whom may develop resistance with YMDD (tyrosine-methionine-aspartate-aspartate) mutant variants of HBV. Entecavir and tenofovir are the typical first-line treatment options in children. Liver transplantation is an effective treatment for children with acute or chronic liver failure, but recurrence is high without prophylaxis.

Table 10-2 lists antiviral drugs that are currently approved by the Food and Drug Administration, only 5 of which are approved for patients younger than 18 years (Evidence Level I).

Table 10-2. Antiviral Therapies for Hepatitis B

Drug	Approved for Children	Resistance
Peginterferon	>1 y for 48 weeks	Not reported
Lamivudine[a]	>2 y	64% after 3 y
Adefovir[b]	>12 y	10% after 2 y
Entecavir	>2 y	Reported
Tenofovir	>12 y	Not reported
Telbivudine	Not approved	—

[a] Not recommended because of a high incidence of resistance.
[b] Not preferred because of weak antiviral activity.

Hepatitis C

Clinical Features

Hepatitis C virus infection is transmitted by contaminated blood or body fluids. The primary mechanism of HCV infection in children is mother-to-infant transmission (vertical transmission). The risk of transmission is 5% to 7% for each pregnancy in an infected mother without concomitant HIV infection and increases by 2-fold to 3-fold with HIV coinfection. High maternal HCV viral load greater than 3,000,000 IU/mL appears to favor mother-to-infant HCV transmission. Chronic HCV is linked to an increased risk of HCC and cirrhosis in adulthood.

About 25% to 40% of infants who acquire HCV by vertical transmission experience spontaneous resolution of the infection by 2 years of age. However, only about 6% to 12% of older children who acquire HCV experience spontaneous resolution.

Most children are clinically asymptomatic. However, in those who develop chronic hepatitis C, the disease is usually progressive, and HCV cirrhosis in children has been reported. Children coinfected with HIV and/or HBV and those who are obese are at an increased risk of developing severe disease (cirrhosis). No good immunizations exist to protect against HCV.

Evaluation

Antibody-based IgG screening tests are automated immunoassays available in most clinical laboratories; they should be performed whenever there is suspicion of HCV infection in a child with unexplained acute liver dysfunction. Hepatitis C virus IgG antibodies are not recommended for screening children younger than 18 months owing to the presence of maternal antibodies. For children in whom there is concern regarding HCV infection, qualitative and quantitative HCV RNA testing and HCV genotyping are used to guide the selection and duration of direct-acting antiviral (DAA) therapy.

Management

Children younger than 3 years typically do not receive antiviral therapy because the chance of spontaneous resolution is high (Evidence Level I). Antiviral therapy is, however, indicated for children with progressive liver disease or advanced histologic features. To date, randomized trials have demonstrated a favorable reduction in viral loads, but there is no evidence of long-term benefit (Evidence Level I). Treatment in children younger than 12 years is typically deferred; however, when an all-oral DAA regimen is available, this will likely change.

Children older than 12 years with genotype 1, 4, 5, or 6 infection receive ledipasvir-sofosbuvir treatment for 12 weeks. Those with genotype 2 or 3 infection are treated with sofosbuvir-velpatasvir in Europe, but this drug is not yet approved in the United States. Sofosbuvir with ribavirin is an alternative, but ribavirin has adverse effects (teratogenicity, anemia). Coinfection with HBV should be eliminated before initiating DAA treatment. Pregnancy should be excluded before beginning treatment with ribavirin. The viral load typically is checked 3 months after the end of treatment to assess the viral response.

HEPATITIS E VIRUS

Hepatitis E virus (HEV) is the most common cause of acute hepatitis in highly endemic areas. Genotypes 1 and 2 are common in endemic countries and are transmitted by means of contaminated water. In Western countries, undercooked pork is the cause of genotype 3 infection (infected swine).

Pregnant women can experience fulminant hepatitis and can vertically transmit HEV to their infants. The virus can also be transmitted through a blood donation from a presymptomatic donor. Infection in immunocompromised hosts (older adults and organ transplant recipients) can lead to chronic hepatitis. Hepatitis E virus–specific anti-IgM and anti-IgG antibody tests are available, and HEV RNA tests can be useful adjuncts. Acute HEV is, for the most part, a self-limited disease. Ribavirin can be used to treat chronic HEV infection in immunocompromised hosts when indicated.

LONG-TERM CONSIDERATIONS

Although each type of viral hepatitis can be associated with fulminant disease to varying degrees (more common with HBV and least common with HAV and HEV), chronic infection and slowly progressive cirrhosis are the more common serious sequelae. Hepatitis B and C virus infections can enter an indolent chronic phase that lasts for years and results in progressive hepatic scarring. It is important to follow children with chronic infection to assess liver function periodically and consider antiviral treatment in those with significant liver involvement. Hepatitis A virus does not appear to be associated with chronic progressive disease, whereas HEV infection causes chronic cirrhosis in immunocompromised hosts.

SUGGESTED READING

American Academy of Pediatrics. *Red Book: 2018–2021 Report of the Committee on Infectious Diseases.* Kimberlin DW, Brady MT, Jackson MA, Long SS, eds. 31st ed. Itasca, IL: American Academy of Pediatrics; 2018

Broderick, A, Jonas MM. Management of hepatitis B virus infection in children and adolescents. UpToDate website. https://www.uptodate.com/contents/management-of-hepatitis-b-virus-infection-in-children-and-adolescents. Updated January 21, 2019. Accessed February 7, 2019

Haber BA, Block JM, Jonas MM, et al. Recommendations for screening, monitoring, and referral of pediatric chronic hepatitis B. *Pediatrics.* 2009;124(5):e1007–e1013

Jakobsen JC, Nielsen EE, Feinberg J, et al. Direct-acting antivirals for chronic hepatitis C. *Cochrane Database Syst Rev.* 2017;9:CD012143

Jonas MM. Hepatitis C virus infection in children. UpToDate website. https://www.uptodate.com/contents/hepatitis-c-virus-infection-in-children. Updated January 16, 2019. Accessed February 7, 2019

Jonas MM, Block JM, Haber BA, et al; Hepatitis B Foundation. Treatment of children with chronic hepatitis B virus infection in the United States: patient selection and therapeutic options. *Hepatology.* 2010;52(6):2192–2205

Mack CL, Gonzalez-Peralta RP, Gupta N, et al; North American Society for Pediatric Gastroenterology, Hepatology, and Nutrition. NASPGHAN practice guidelines: diagnosis and management of hepatitis C infection in infants, children, and adolescents. *J Pediatr Gastroenterol Nutr.* 2012;54(6):838–855

Mantzoukis K, Rodríguez-Perálvarez M, Buzzetti E, et al. Pharmacological interventions for acute hepatitis B infection: an attempted network meta-analysis. *Cochrane Database Syst Rev.* 2017;3:CD011645

Hepatosplenomegaly

Toba A. Weinstein, MD

OVERVIEW

Hepatosplenomegaly, the simultaneous enlargement of both the liver and spleen, is always a pathologic finding. Hepatomegaly is a valuable marker of liver disease, even without accompanying splenomegaly. Organ enlargement occurs via 5 general mechanisms: as a result of inflammation, infiltration, abnormal storage, congestion, or obstruction. Although hepatosplenomegaly is most commonly caused by an infectious process, the presence of an enlarged liver and spleen may be the first sign of an underlying metabolic, hematologic, or malignant disorder.

A palpable liver is not always a sign of hepatomegaly. Although a liver edge that is palpable more than 2 cm below the right costal margin at the midclavicular line is suggestive of liver enlargement, hepatomegaly is only present when there is an increase in total liver span. Newborns, on average, have a normal liver span of approximately 5 cm, a measurement that increases with age, with adolescents having an average liver span of between 6 and 8 cm.

Anatomic variations in the liver may also cause a clinician to suspect hepatomegaly. Riedel lobe is a downward, tongue-like projection of the right lobe of the liver that may give the false impression of hepatomegaly on imaging.

Although a spleen tip may be palpable in up to 5% of children, the presence of hepatosplenomegaly on physical examination is always a concerning clinical finding that necessitates further evaluation.

CAUSES AND DIFFERENTIAL DIAGNOSIS

The causes of hepatosplenomegaly in infants and children are shown in **Box 11-1**. Cholestasis associated with hepatosplenomegaly suggests an infection, portal hypertension, or an extramedullary hematopoiesis as a potential etiology, with metabolic disorders and congenital infections being the more common etiologies during the neonatal period.

Box 11-1. Differential Diagnosis of Hepatosplenomegaly

Infections
- Viral
  - Congenital
    - Cytomegalovirus
    - Epstein-Barr virus
    - Enterovirus
    - Herpes simplex
    - Rubella
  - Hepatitis A, B, and C
  - HIV
- Bacterial
  - Bacterial liver abscess
  - Subacute bacterial endocarditis
  - *Bartonella*
  - Brucellosis
  - Congenital syphilis
  - Tuberculosis
- Parasitic
  - Leishmaniasis
  - Malaria
  - Schistosomiasis
  - Toxoplasmosis
- Fungal
  - Candidiasis
  - Histoplasmosis
  - Coccidioidomycosis

Metabolic diseases and genetic disorders
- Glycogen storage disease
  - Andersen disease
- Lysosomal storage disorders
  - Cholesterol ester storage disease
  - Gaucher disease
  - Hurler syndrome
  - Niemann-Pick disease
  - Sandhoff disease
  - Wolman disease
- Disorders of amino acid metabolism
  - Tyrosinemia
- Disorders of carbohydrate metabolism
  - Galactosemia
- Other genetic disorders
  - Cystic fibrosis

Malignant and hematologic disorders
- Histiocytosis
- Leukemia
- Lymphoma
- Neuroblastoma

▼▲▼▲▼▲▼▲▼▲▼▲▼▲▼   ▲▼▲▼▲▼▲▼▲▼▲▼▲▼▲▼

Box 11-1. Differential Diagnosis of Hepatosplenomegaly (*continued*)

Hepatic and Congestive Processes

Portal hypertension
  Congestive heart failure
  Restrictive pericarditis
  Budd-Chiari syndrome
  Veno-occlusive disease
Biliary obstruction
  Extrahepatic biliary
    atresia

Systemic Inflammatory Disorders

Inflammatory bowel
  disease
Juvenile rheumatoid
  arthritis
Sarcoidosis
Systemic lupus
  erythematosus

Infection

Infection, particularly viral infection, is the most common cause of hepato-splenomegaly in the pediatric population. Infectious mononucleosis secondary to the Epstein-Barr virus is the most common infectious cause of an enlarged spleen in an adolescent in developed countries. Children with hepatitis A, B, and C can have isolated hepatomegaly as well as hepatosplenomegaly. If multiple hepatic abscesses are noted, an immunodeficiency such as chronic granulomatous disease or severe combined immunodeficiency should be considered. Parasitic infections are less common in developed countries than in developing countries. Fungal infections are rare in immunocompetent patients. Hepatosplenic involvement typically results from seeding during generalized fungemia in immunosuppressed individuals. Candidiasis, histoplasmosis, and coccidioidomycosis can develop in immunocompromised children with the appropriate exposure.

Metabolic and Genetic Disorders

Cholestasis in association with hepatosplenomegaly in an infant without a congenital infection or sepsis strongly suggests an underlying metabolic or genetic disorder. These disorders include storage disease and enzyme deficiencies. In the older child, lysosomal storage disorders are the most common metabolic cause of hepatosplenomegaly. Lysosomal storage disorders are a group of rare genetic enzyme deficiencies, and hepatosplenomegaly is a clinical manifestation in several of them. These disorders include cholesterol ester storage disease, Gaucher disease, Hurler syndrome, Niemann-Pick disease, Sandhoff disease, and Wolman disease. Gaucher disease is the most common metabolic cause of hepatosplenomegaly in older children, and it results from an accumulation of glucocerebrosides in the cells of the reticuloendothelial system. In Hurler syndrome, hepatosplenomegaly develops during the first year after birth. Neimann-Pick disease is always associated with hepatosplenomegaly. Neonates with Wolman disease develop failure to thrive, cholestasis, and hepatosplenomegaly shortly after birth and often have adrenal calcifications, and their condition continues to worsen over time. Cholesterol ester storage disease is a milder disorder, with hepatomegaly or hepatosplenomegaly occurring later in life.

Type IV glycogen storage disease (Andersen disease) is associated with hepatosplenomegaly and failure to thrive during infancy. Infants with tyrosinemia may present with acute liver failure and severe hepatic synthetic dysfunction in addition to hepatosplenomegaly. Hepatobiliary disease can occur in up to one-half of all patients with cystic fibrosis.

Malignant and Hematologic Disorders

Infants and children with myeloproliferative and lymphoproliferative disorders can develop hepatosplenomegaly. Acute lymphoblastic leukemia often presents with bone and joint pain in addition to fever, hepatosplenomegaly, and lymphadenopathy. Patients with metastatic neoplastic disease such as lymphoma, neuroblastoma, and histiocytosis also can develop hepatosplenomegaly. Hemophagocytic lymphohistiocytosis can occur with hepatosplenomegaly, with resultant fulminant hepatic failure and its associated morbidity and mortality.

Hepatic and Congestive Processes

Hepatic congestion may develop if venous outflow from the liver is impeded. Portal hypertension with increased portal venous pressure and associated splenomegaly can develop in patients without cirrhosis. Suprahepatic portal hypertension may result from restrictive pericardial disease, congestive heart failure, or Budd-Chiari syndrome. Doppler studies are particularly useful to assess for vein thrombosis. Patients with veno-occlusive disease also can develop hepatosplenomegaly. This involvement of the small veins in the liver can be seen in patients after transplantation or in children who are receiving certain chemotherapeutic agents.

Extrahepatic biliary atresia may manifest as hepatosplenomegaly and should be strongly considered in a healthy newborn who gradually develops hepatosplenomegaly in association with failure to thrive, cholestasis, and acholic stools between 1 and 3 months of age. This finding is a result of bile flow obstruction. It is one of the most common conditions that leads to the need for liver transplantation in childhood.

CLINICAL FEATURES

Patients with hepatosplenomegaly are often asymptomatic; however, they may complain of right upper quadrant pain. Abdominal distention or abdominal protuberance may be reported as a symptom or noted on the physical examination. Gastrointestinal symptoms such as abdominal pain, nausea, vomiting, and diarrhea may occur. These findings are most common in patients with infectious, metabolic, or systemic disorders. Patients with infectious causes may develop a fever. Other individuals may have jaundice and scleral icterus. Features associated with cholestasis such as a change in urine and/or stool color also may be reported by the patient or caregiver.

Failure to thrive, weight loss, and anorexia are also common symptoms in neonates and children with hepatosplenomegaly. Some individuals have a bleeding diathesis as a result of thrombocytopenia secondary to sequestration from splenomegaly or due to another coagulopathy related to an underlying liver dysfunction.

EVALUATION

Imaging Studies

An abdominal radiograph can suggest the presence of hepatosplenomegaly, and often an enlarged liver and spleen may be an incidental finding on a radiographic study. Calcifications noted on abdominal radiographs can be located in the liver, spleen, biliary tree, or vasculature. Calcification may be a sign of malignancy, portal vein thrombosis, or parasitic infection. If calcification is noted, the physician should promptly order further radiographic imaging. Abdominal ultrasonography should be the first imaging study ordered when evaluating a patient for hepatosplenomegaly. Combined with doppler flow imaging, ultrasonography can help in the evaluation of blood flow, including patency of the hepatic and portal vein and collateral circulation.

Computed tomography (CT) and magnetic resonance imaging (MRI) can detect focal lesions including tumors, cysts, and abscesses. Abdominal CT is the best method to define the extent of solid or cystic lesions, as well as the vascularity of hepatic or splenic lesions (Evidence Level III). Magnetic resonance imaging is an excellent tool for the diagnosis and evaluation of focal lesions and pathologic conditions of the liver and particularly the spleen in patients with splenomegaly. The large fractional heme content of the spleen underlies the benefit of MRI, which provides excellent resolution without radiation; however, sedation is often required in the younger child.

Radionuclide scanning is used to assess hepatic and splenic function. Scans also can help detect focal lesions such as tumors, cysts, or abscesses but they lack the resolution of CT or MRI.

Laboratory Evaluation

Laboratory evaluation (**Box 11-2**) can be beneficial in the assessment of infants and children with hepatosplenomegaly. Certain components of a complete blood cell count (CBC) may be affected by a massively enlarged spleen. Although the white blood cell count (WBC) is typically elevated in patients with an infectious process, the WBC may be normal or decreased in children

Box 11-2. Initial Laboratory Evaluation for Hepatosplenomegaly

- Complete blood cell count
- Liver-related enzymes
  - Aspartate aminotransferase
  - Alanine aminotransferase
  - Alkaline phosphatase
  - γ-Glutamyltransferase
  - Bilirubin (total and fractionated)
  - Albumin
- Coagulation profile
  - Prothrombin time
  - International normalized ratio
  - Partial thromboplastin time

or infants with massive splenomegaly secondary to splenic sequestration. Likewise, patients with significant splenomegaly may have thrombocytopenia due to splenic sequestration. Although the platelet count, which is an acute-phase reactant, may be elevated, it is typically normal or low in patients with hepatosplenomegaly. The most marked transaminase elevation occurs with acute hepatocellular injury. Transaminase elevation may develop with or without cholestasis. Clinicians may observe elevated transaminase levels in infants and children with hepatomegaly secondary to infection, infiltration, and/or an underlying metabolic disease or systemic process. In addition, albumin, prothrombin time, and international normalized ratio measurements aid in the assessment of synthetic liver function (Evidence Level III).

Other laboratory investigations may be indicated, such as an assessment for congenital infections including toxoplasmosis, rubella, cytomegalovirus, herpes, HIV, syphilis, and other hepatitides in the neonate, as well as an assessment for bacterial infection and sepsis. In the older child, a laboratory evaluation for infectious mononucleosis and hepatitis should be performed.

When a metabolic disorder is suspected, further evaluation is needed, including serum glucose, ketones, lactate, pyruvate, and ammonia levels, as well as evaluation of urine for organic acids and serum for amino acids. In addition, evaluation of specific enzyme markers should be tailored to the specific patient.

If the physician suspects a malignant process, he or she should test for alpha-fetoprotein levels, which can suggest malignancy such as hepatoma, hepatoblastoma, or hereditary tyrosinemia.

Biopsy

Sometimes a biopsy must be performed to obtain tissue for microscopic, enzymatic, and/or genetic testing in infants and children with hepatosplenomegaly to help elucidate the underlying disease process. The type of tissue specimen obtained for pathologic evaluation is based on the clinical, laboratory, and radiographic findings of hepatosplenomegaly.

The results of a liver biopsy may suggest an etiology for hepatomegaly in patients with hepatocellular injury or cholestatic disease; a liver biopsy also is extremely helpful in evaluating patients in whom the cause of their chronic hepatitis or underlying metabolic disorder is unknown (Evidence Level III). A liver biopsy can be performed percutaneously, but in high-risk patients, this procedure may best be performed by a surgeon or an interventional radiologist.

Lymph node biopsy results may suggest an etiology for hepatosplenomegaly in patients in whom a malignant or an infectious process is strongly considered based on the results of laboratory and radiographic testing. A pediatric surgeon typically performs this procedure and sends the tissue for appropriate culture and pathologic evaluation.

A bone marrow biopsy, performed by a hematologist, may be required when a hematologic or malignant process is suspected in a child with hepatosplenomegaly. Less commonly, an organ-specific biopsy, such as a skin or muscle biopsy, may be necessary, with the tissue specimen tested to help identify a metabolic etiology in a patient with hepatosplenomegaly.

MANAGEMENT

Supportive care should be provided in all cases. Treatment must be individualized based on disease presentation and the eventual diagnosis. However, the earlier the cause of hepatosplenomegaly is determined, the more rapidly that treatment can be initiated.

Most patients with acute viral infections, such as those with infectious mononucleosis, respond well to supportive care only (Evidence Level III). Antiviral therapy is seldom initiated. Bacterial, parasitic, and fungal infections are treated with antibiotics and antiparasitic and antifungal medications, with the treatment course and duration tailored to the offending pathogen.

Treatment of patients with underlying hematologic and malignant disorders often entails a chemotherapeutic regimen. Adjuvant surgery or radiation therapy also may be required. Patients with metabolic or genetic disorders may need enzyme replacement therapy, as well as medication and a possible dietary intervention.

LONG-TERM MONITORING

Hepatosplenomegaly resolves in most patients who present with acute viral infections, although a subset with hepatitis may require antiviral therapy. These individuals should be closely monitored. A hematologist or an oncologist also needs to closely monitor children with underlying hematologic or malignant disorders.

▼△▼△▼△▼△▼△▼△▼△▼△▼ ▼△▼△▼△▼△▼△▼△▼△▼△▼

SUGGESTED READING

Baker A. Hepatosplenomegaly. *Paediatr Child Health*. 2017;27(5):247–249

Clayton PT. Inborn errors presenting with liver dysfunction. *Semin Neonatol*. 2002;7(1):49–63

Konus OL, Ozdemir A, Akkaya A, et al. Normal liver, spleen, and kidney dimensions in neonates, infants and children: evaluation with sonography. *Am J Roentgenol*. 1998;171(6):1693–1698

Megremis SD, Vlachonikolis IG, Tsilimigaki AM. Spleen length in childhood with US: normal values based on age, sex, and somatometric parameters. *Radiology*. 2004;231(1):129–134

Wolf AD, Lavine JE. Hepatomegaly in neonates and children. *Pediatr Rev*. 2000;21(9):303–310

Hirschsprung Disease and Other Gastrointestinal Motility Disorders

Meenakshi Rao, MD, PhD, and Samuel Nurko, MD, MPH

OVERVIEW

Gastrointestinal (GI) motility disorders in children are common and range from
benign conditions, such as gastroesophageal reflux and functional constipation
to others that cause significant morbidity and mortality, such as Hirschsprung
disease (HD) and chronic intestinal pseudo-obstruction. Dysmotility can
affect any segment of the GI tract and trigger a variety of symptoms, including
dysphagia, abdominal pain, abdominal distention, and fecal incontinence.
Figure 12-1 presents a general algorithm for the approach to a child with
a suspected GI motility disorder. With any suspected motility disorder, it is
imperative to first rule out an anatomic obstruction and then determine if there
is a problem with GI transit. Motility testing is often indicated to demonstrate
abnormal patterns of motility and to delineate underlying pathophysiology.
Once a diagnosis of dysmotility is made, it is important to determine whether it
represents a primary motility disorder (eg, achalasia, HD, pseudo-obstruction)
or is secondary to a systemic disorder (eg, mitochondrial disease). For a child
with a motility disorder, providing supportive care is essential to maintain adequate nutrition, manage pain, avoid common complications such as intestinal
bacterial overgrowth, and decompress obstructed bowel segments when needed.
Interventions for bowel decompression in children with severe dysmotility can
range from placing venting gastrostomy tubes to surgical procedures such as
ileostomy. In addition to describing the general approach to managing a child
with signs and/or symptoms of a GI motility disorder, this chapter focuses on

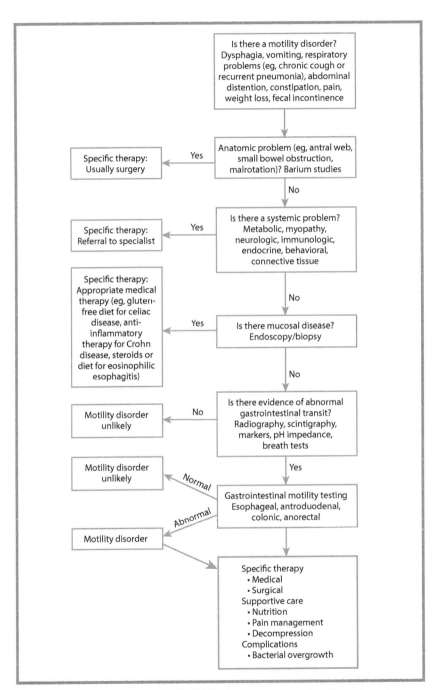

Figure 12-1. Approach to the Child With a Suspected Motility Disorder

2 distinct motility disorders—HD and gastroparesis—to elucidate specific evaluation and management approaches.

HIRSCHSPRUNG DISEASE

Beyond the neonatal period, chronic idiopathic constipation is the most frequent cause of childhood constipation (see **Chapter 5**). In rare cases, however, constipation can be caused by primary motor abnormalities, such as HD or congenital megacolon. Diagnosing HD is important because of the risks and need for specific treatment.

Causes

Hirschsprung disease is a defect in colonization of the intestine by the enteric nervous system during embryonic development. In 90% of patients with HD, only the rectosigmoid colon is involved. Five percent of patients have total colonic aganglionosis. Approximately 15% of patients with HD have at least 1 other congenital anomaly. The genetic syndromes associated most commonly with HD are listed in **Box 12-1.**

Differential Diagnosis

In an infant or a young child with signs and/or symptoms of a GI motility disorder, functional constipation (chronic idiopathic constipation) is important to consider. A number of anatomic GI tract disorders such as anorectal malformations, internal anal sphincter achalasia, small left colon (associated with maternal diabetes), and colonic atresia are also part of the differential diagnosis in these children. In the newborn, meconium ileus causes significant bowel dysfunction and is pathognomonic for cystic fibrosis. In children of all ages, hypothyroidism and severe electrolyte disturbances (hypokalemia, hyponatremia) can also lead to bowel dysmotility.

Clinical Features

Most children with HD are diagnosed in the neonatal period, when failure to pass meconium within 48 hours of birth is the presenting sign. Notable presenting symptoms include abdominal distention, vomiting, and inability to tolerate oral feedings. While 99% of full-term infants without HD pass meconium within the first 48 hours of birth, only 30% of newborns with HD pass meconium during this period. Thus, failure to pass meconium within 48 hours should raise concern for HD. Some infants with HD present later in childhood with fulminant diarrhea, fever, and sepsis-like physiology characteristic of Hirschsprung-associated enterocolitis (HAEC), which may be the first sign in up to 12% of

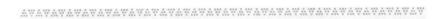

Box 12-1. Genetic Syndromes Associated With Hirschsprung Disease (HD)

- Trisomy 21 (2% to 3% of patients with HD)
- Bardet-Biedl syndrome
- Cartilage-hair hypoplasia
- Congenital central hypoventilation syndrome (20% of patients have HD)
- Multiple endocrine neoplasia type 2
- Mowat-Wilson syndrome (50% of patients have HD)
- Waardenburg syndrome
- Congenital heart disease
- Renal or genitourinary abnormalities

patients. Enterocolitis continues to be the principal cause of death in cases of HD. From infancy though adulthood, constipation may be the only presenting symptom. Clinical characteristics alone do not always distinguish HD from functional constipation; therefore, clinicians should consider HD in all patients with intractable constipation.

EVALUATION

Physical Examination

Frequent physical examination findings in children with HD include abdominal distention, tight anal canal on digital rectal examination (DRE), and the classic "squirt sign"—explosive release of fecal contents on DRE.

Diagnostic Studies

Plain abdominal radiographs (kidneys, ureter, bladder [KUB]) are typically obtained in evaluation of the infant or child with signs of abdominal distension and/or dysmotility (Evidence Level III). The presence of dilated bowel loops

▼▲▼▲▼▲▼▲▼▲▼▲▼▲▼ ▼ ▲▼▲▼▲▼▲▼▲▼▲▼▲▼▲▼

with no air in the rectum is consistent with distal intestinal obstruction and suggests HD. More concerning findings such as widespread air fluid levels, proximal colonic distention, and an abrupt cutoff of luminal air at the pelvic brim are all strongly suggestive of HAEC. In a child older than 3 months who is suspected of having HD, the test of choice is anorectal manometry, which evaluates internal anal sphincter relaxation after balloon distention. In patients with HD, sphincter relaxation is not present and indicates the need to perform a rectal biopsy for definitive diagnosis. Anorectal manometry is very sensitive and specific in children older than 3 months, and normal findings mean that a rectal biopsy is not needed. Disadvantages of this test are that it may require sedation in young children and is typically available only in specialized institutions.

The gold standard for diagnosing HD is demonstration of the absence of enteric ganglion cells on rectal suction or full-thickness biopsy. Rectal suction biopsies are usually performed without the need for anesthesia or sedation. Primary risks are bleeding, intestinal perforation, and inadequate tissue sampling. Histologic findings of absent ganglion cells and hypertrophic nerve fibers, as well as increased acetylcholinesterase activity are characteristics of HD (Evidence Level III). For infants younger than 3 months, the rectal suction biopsy is the most sensitive and specific test for HD. A full-thickness rectal biopsy may be required to establish a diagnosis of HD if a rectal suction biopsy is indeterminate as a result of inadequate tissue sampling. A full-thickness rectal biopsy is also performed intraoperatively during surgical repair in patients with known HD to identify the transition zone from ganglionic to aganglionic intestine.

A contrast enema is a radiographic study that can be obtained for evaluation of suspected HD. In HD, this study reveals a distinct transition zone between the narrowed aganglionic segment and proximal dilated bowel. The surgeon often uses a barium enema for preoperative planning in children with HD. It is important to recognize that this test can be falsely negative in neonates following DRE or rectal irrigation, which relieve the obstruction. A normal barium enema in a newborn with bilious vomiting and no evidence of malrotation still points to HD until the rectal suction biopsy proves otherwise.

MANAGEMENT

Surgery is the definitive therapy for HD and consists of resection of the aganglionic segment, pull-through of the proximal unaffected segment, and anastomosis to the distal segment to bring bowel into continuity.

Appropriate preoperative and postoperative care is essential to minimize the occurrence of HAEC and optimize defecatory function. Frequent loose stools are common during the early postoperative period as the bowel adapts. Avoiding hypertonic phosphate enemas in patients with known or suspected HD is important because prolonged bowel retention can lead to significant electrolyte abnormalities.

Patients with possible HAEC can be treated on an outpatient basis with oral metronidazole and oral hydration with an electrolyte-rich solution. Rectal irrigations to wash out retained stool from the colon may relieve abdominal distension. In more severe cases of definitive HAEC, patients are hospitalized and treated with clear liquids or intravenous fluids to provide bowel rest. Nasogastric decompression may be needed if abdominal distension is significant. Rectal irrigation is often used to resolve fecal stasis. Metronidazole (oral or parenteral) is used to treat anaerobes, including *Clostridium difficile*, which has been associated with HAEC. In addition to metronidazole, broad-spectrum intravenous antibiotic coverage often is used, with a combination of ampicillin and gentamicin, piperacillin/tazobactam, or aztreonam (in the case of penicillin allergy) (Evidence Level III). In fact, 4 weeks of probiotic therapy has been shown to decrease the incidence and severity of HAEC in children (Evidence Level I).

LONG-TERM MONITORING

Although most patients with HD achieve bowel continence over time, the prevalence of defecation disorders, including constipation, fecal soiling, and increased stool frequency, is high. Notably, patients with HD remain at lifelong risk for enterocolitis despite having undergone surgical removal of the aganglionic segment; the incidence is as high as 30% of all children with HD (Evidence Level III). Patients may experience progression of aganglionosis to unaffected segments or develop anastomotic strictures, leading to obstructive symptoms. Strictures may be treated with anal dilations, botulinum toxin, and antibiotic therapy for bacterial overgrowth.

GASTROPARESIS

OVERVIEW

Gastroparesis is delayed gastric emptying in the absence of a mechanical outlet obstruction.

CAUSES

Most cases of gastroparesis in children are idiopathic, although there are secondary causes, especially in children with chronic medical conditions (**Box 12-2**).

Box 12-2. Causes of Gastroparesis in Children

Idiopathic

Postinfectious (usually viral infection)

Postsurgical
- Percutaneous endoscopic gastrostomy
- Nissen fundoplication

Endocrine disorders
- Diabetes mellitus
- Hypothyroidism

Prematurity

Inflammatory (Crohn disease or eosinophilic gastroenteropathy)

Metabolic derangement
- Hypokalemia
- Acidosis

Neuromuscular disorders
- Muscular dystrophy
- Cerebral palsy
- Chronic intestinal pseudo-obstruction

Medications
- Opioids
- Anticholinergics
- Anticonvulsants

▼▲▼▲▼▲▼▲▼▲▼▲▼▲▼▲▼   ▼▲▼▲▼▲▼▲▼▲▼▲▼▲▼▲▼

DIFFERENTIAL DIAGNOSIS

In a child with gastroparesis, the search for an underlying disorder will usually be unsuccessful. Anatomic abnormalities of the esophagus and stomach, such as gastroesophageal reflux, achalasia, and antral web, are important considerations. Intestinal obstruction is a serious cause of gastroparesis that must be excluded, particularly if no stomach abnormality is defined. Rumination in the younger child and eating disorders such as bulimia in older children and adolescents are important psychogenic causes of gastroparesis.

CLINICAL FEATURES

Vomiting and abdominal pain are the most common symptoms of gastroparesis. Other symptoms include nausea, weight loss, early satiety, and bloating. Vomiting is usually postprandial, frequently contains undigested food, and typically occurs 30 minutes or more after a meal. In these children, liquids are typically easier to tolerate than solids. In contrast, patients with esophageal disorders rather than gastric dysmotility typically complain of dysphagia, regurgitation, and vomiting immediately after oral intake. Bilious emesis should raise concern for a mechanical obstruction such as intestinal malrotation. Postviral gastroparesis may be the most common identifiable etiology in children. It is often suggested by a history of fevers, myalgias, nausea, or diarrhea occurring before presentation and usually is a self-limited disorder.

EVALUATION

Physical Examination

The physical examination findings are normal in idiopathic gastroparesis, but children with secondary disorders may have distinct abnormalities (see **Box 12-2**). Signs of malnutrition and/or a markedly distended abdomen may underscore a secondary cause of gastroparesis.

Diagnostic Evaluation

A common finding in plain abdominal radiographs (ie, KUB) in the child with gastroparesis is a large gastric bubble. More specific abnormalities such as a radiodense foreign body also may be detected. An upper GI (UGI) barium study is an important diagnostic step that can help rule out gastric bezoars, intestinal malrotation, and antral webs. A UGI study can also identify rare causes of gastroparesis, such as achalasia, that may have some overlap in presentation.

Several laboratory tests, including thyroid function tests, electrolyte panels, and celiac serologic tests, can be useful in searching for secondary causes of vomiting, abdominal distension, and gastroparesis.

If the initial workup reveals no evidence of a mechanical obstruction or secondary causes of gastroparesis, initiating first-line therapies without further diagnostic testing is a reasonable course (see Management section). Additional diagnostic studies can establish the presence of delayed gastric emptying as a partial cause of such symptoms. Gastric emptying nuclide scintigraphy permits calculation of the efficiency of gastric emptying. Its advantages include minimal radiation exposure, noninvasive nature, and approximation of a typical meal volume. Some disadvantages include challenges in deciding the content of the study meal, timing of imaging, and the center-to-center variability in data reporting. No normative data are available for children; therefore, results must be interpreted with caution. Furthermore, the extent of delayed emptying does not correlate with the degree of symptoms. In adults, consensus standards based on intake of a low-fat egg white meal define delayed gastric emptying as gastric retention of more than 70% at 2 hours or more than 10% at 4 hours. The diagnostic utility of this study is that if the rate of solid meal emptying from the stomach is rapid via nuclear scintigraphy, then a diagnosis of gastroparesis is unlikely.

Antroduodenal manometry often requires sedation for setup; as the child recovers from sedation, pressure measurements from the gastric antrum and duodenum are obtained during fasting, with ingestion of meal, and in response to promotility agents such as erythromycin and octreotide. Although this study can provide extensive information about the biomechanics of gastric emptying and patients' response to medications, it is invasive and requires sedation or anesthesia and a prolonged period of observation. A thorough study also requires some degree of patient cooperation. This study can identify postviral gastroparesis, which demonstrates antral hypomotility and normal duodenal motility; neuropathic conditions, which demonstrate normal amplitude contractions with abnormal or uncoordinated propagation; and myopathic conditions, which demonstrate well-coordinated but low-amplitude contractions. In the future, a wireless motility capsule may become more widely used to define gastric motility and responsiveness in children.

MANAGEMENT

Treatment of gastroparesis is mostly supportive, with a goal of maintaining nutrition and improving gastric function, unless a secondary cause is identified. In children with a secondary cause, specific interventions, such as surgery, are often warranted. Patients with idiopathic gastroparesis should be advised to eat smaller, more frequent meals that are low in fat because high-fat meals slow gastric emptying. In some cases, postpyloric nutritional supplementation may be necessary. Antiemetics are often used to control nausea (Evidence Level II). Prokinetic drugs designed to improve gastric emptying in children include erythromycin, metoclopramide, domperidone, and cisapride. The Food and Drug Administration has assigned a black box warning to metoclopramide owing to neurologic long-term side effects, while both domperidone and cisapride are unavailable in the United States. The drugs detailed in **Table 12-1** are more commonly used.

Table 12-1. Commonly Used Therapeutic Agents for Gastroparesis

Drug (Mechanism of Action)	Dosing	Side Effects
Erythromycin (motilin agonist, accelerates gastric emptying and stimulates small bowel contractions)	3 mg/kg/dose orally or intravenously every 8 h Maximum dose: 250 mg	Abdominal cramping, medication interactions (eg, anticonvulsants)
Cyproheptadine (antihistamine, promotes gastric accommodation; useful as adjunctive therapy but not as monotherapy)	0.25 mg/kg divided twice/d Maximum daily dose: 2–6 y: 12 mg ≥7 y: 16 mg	Drowsiness, appetite stimulation

Other: Injection of botulinum toxin into the pylorus has been successful in children (Evidence Level II).
Gastric pacing: used in a limited number of pediatric patients (Evidence Level II).

LONG-TERM MONITORING

Most children with idiopathic or postviral gastroparesis eventually recover normal gastric emptying function. In the interim, medications such as erythromycin can be helpful in relieving symptoms. Both erythromycin and cyproheptadine can lose efficacy over time as patients develop tachyphylaxis. This problem can be addressed by cycling off the medication for 1 week of every 4 to 6 weeks. Children with severe functional compromise, such as malnutrition, or have lengthy school absences, as well as those who do not respond to first-line therapy, should be referred to a pediatric gastroenterologist for further evaluation.

SUGGESTED READING

Amiel J, Sproat-Emison E, Garcia-Barcelo M, et al; Hirschsprung Disease Consortium. Hirschsprung disease, associated syndromes and genetics: a review. *J Med Genet.* 2008;45(1):1–14

Camilleri M, Parkman HP, Shafi MA, Abell TL, Gerson L; American College of Gastroenterology. Clinical guideline: management of gastroparesis. *Am J Gastroenterol.* 2013;108(1):18–38

Chumpitazi B, Nurko S. Pediatric gastrointestinal motility disorders: challenges and a clinical update. *Gastroenterol Hepatol (N Y).* 2008;4(2):140–148

Gosain A, Frykman PK, Cowles RA, et al; American Pediatric Surgical Association Hirschsprung Disease Interest Group. Guidelines for the diagnosis and management of Hirschsprung-associated enterocolitis. *Pediatr Surg Int.* 2017;33(5):517–521

Langer JC, Rollins MD, Levitt M, et al; American Pediatric Surgical Association Hirschsprung Disease Interest Group. Guidelines for the management of postoperative obstructive symptoms in children with Hirschsprung disease. *Pediatr Surg Int.* 2017;33(5):523–526

Rintala RJ, Pakarinen MP. Long-term outcomes of Hirschsprung's disease. *Semin Pediatr Surg.* 2012;21(4):336–343

Waseem S, Islam S, Kahn G, Moshiree B, Talley NJ. Spectrum of gastroparesis in children. *J Pediatr Gastroenterol Nutr.* 2012;55(2):166–172

Inflammatory Bowel Diseases

Victor M. Piñeiro, MD

OVERVIEW

Inflammatory bowel disease (IBD) encompasses several conditions that are characterized by chronic or relapsing inflammation of the gastrointestinal (GI) tract. Crohn disease (CD) and ulcerative colitis (UC) are the 2 most common distinct subtypes of IBD. A third, less common, subtype, IBD unclassified, may be seen in up to 10% of pediatric patients. Crohn disease is the most common subtype in children, with an incidence of more than twice that of UC. About 25% of patients with IBD present before 20 years of age, most commonly in early adolescence. Although rare, children younger than 5 years who develop IBD may have more aggressive disease and be difficult to treat. The symptoms vary widely at the time of presentation, ranging from insidious growth failure in an otherwise asymptomatic child to a child with fulminant colitis with profuse bloody diarrhea.

CAUSES

Although the exact etiology of IBD is unclear, available evidence points to a complex interaction of genetic predisposition, host immune factors, the patient's intestinal florae (microbiome), and environmental influences. The single greatest risk factor for the development of IBD is having a first degree relative with the diagnosis. Since the first IBD gene (*NOD2*) was identified in 2001, there has been an exponential increase in the number of defined genetic risk factors for IBD. The complex interaction of intestinal mucosal immune mechanisms with the patient's microbiome is thought to be critical in the development of IBD. Proposed mechanisms include an appropriate response to a persistent pathogenic infection or an inappropriate response to the patient's microbiome. Multiple altered immune mechanisms have also been proposed as possible causes of IBD. Proposed factors include a defective barrier function, which may lead to increased permeability to bacterial antigens, or a defective immune response, which could lead to the state of chronic inflammation seen in IBD.

SIGNS AND SYMPTOMS

The initial presentation of IBD can vary depending on the extent of GI tract involvement, severity of the inflammatory process, presence of GI strictures, and/or extraintestinal manifestations. Crohn disease can affect any part of the intestinal tract, most frequently the distal ileum and the cecum, whereas UC affects only the colon. In CD, the inflammation tends to be segmental, with skip areas (regions of normal bowel between inflamed areas). In CD, small bowel disease is often obstructive, usually in the distal ileum, causing right lower quadrant pain. Colonic CD and UC most often present with symptoms of colitis (diarrhea, tenesmus, bleeding, and cramping). Ulcerative colitis is localized to the colon and spares the upper GI tract any inflammatory involvement (although mild chronic gastritis can be observed). Ulcerative colitis usually begins in the rectum and extends proximally. Approximately 50% to 80% of pediatric patients with UC have extensive colitis (pancolitis).

It is usually possible to distinguish between UC and CD by the clinical presentation, disease extent, and radiographic, endoscopic, and histopathologic findings (**tables 13-1** and **13-2**). Overall, extraintestinal manifestations occur more frequently in CD than in UC (see **Table 13-2**).

EVALUATION

Patients with abdominal pain and colitis symptoms (diarrhea, tenesmus, and blood in the stool) are usually diagnosed earlier than patients with chronic abdominal pain or growth failure. The subtle and insidious onset of symptoms in CD may lead to 1- to 2-year delay before a final diagnosis is made, whereas children with UC are often diagnosed sooner. The physical examination findings listed in **Table 13-3** are compatible with a diagnosis of IBD. The presence of any of these findings should raise suspicion for IBD. Basic laboratory and stool studies can assist in the diagnosis (**Box 13-1**).

The diagnosis of IBD must be confirmed by endoscopic and histologic examination of the esophagus, stomach, duodenum, and colon. Given the importance of differentiating between UC and CD, most patients with suspected IBD require endoscopic and imaging evaluation of the upper GI tract and the small bowel in addition to a colonoscopy (Evidence Level III). Imaging studies

Table 13-1. Clinical Features of Crohn Disease and Ulcerative Colitis

Feature	Crohn Disease (% of patients)	Ulcerative Colitis (% of patients)
Abdominal pain	75	85
Diarrhea	65	90
Rectal bleeding	20	90
Weight loss	65	50
Growth retardation	15–40	Less common
Perianal disease	25	Rare
Nausea/vomiting	25	25
Nocturnal diarrhea	Less common	50
Oral ulcerations	20	Less common

to assess the colon are rarely needed given the safety and specificity of colonoscopy. However, imaging studies are needed to assess the small bowel. Computed tomographic or magnetic resonance (MR) enterography can be performed to visualize the small bowel; nevertheless, MR enterography is preferred to avoid radiation exposure (Evidence Level II-2). Video capsule endoscopy can be performed in the cooperative child when there is doubt about the diagnosis of UC versus CD, as well as to follow disease activity over time.

Children with IBD are at high risk for osteopenia. Dual-energy x-ray absorptiometry (DEXA) is the preferred screening tool for children and adolescents with IBD (Evidence Level II-2). The current consensus recommendation is to obtain a DEXA scan of the spine and total body at presentation or at any point in children with IBD and any of the following risk factors: suboptimal growth velocity, downward crossing height percentile curves, weight or body mass index z score less than −2.0 standard deviations, secondary or primary amenorrhea, delayed puberty, severe inflammatory disease course, continuous use of systemic glucocorticoids for 6 or more months (Evidence Level II-2).

Table 13-2. Extraintestinal Manifestations and Extent of Disease in Crohn Disease and Ulcerative Colitis

Feature	Crohn Disease (% of patients)	Ulcerative Colitis (% of patients)
Joint symptoms	Present (30–40)	Present (30)
Pyoderma gangrenosum	Rare (1–2)	Rare (1–2)
Erythema nodosum	Present (10)	Less common (2–4)
Sclerosing cholangitis	Less common	Present (3–4)
Thrombosis	Less common	Present
Rectal involvement	Occasional	Always
Colonic disease	50–75	100
Ileal disease	Common (50–60)	Occasional backwash ileitis
Gastroduodenal disease	Present (30)	Chronic gastritis (30)
Strictures	Common	Rare
Fissures	Common	Rare
Perianal fistulas	Common	Rare
Toxic megacolon	None	Present
Cancer risk	Increased	Greatly increased

DIFFERENTIAL DIAGNOSIS

The protean manifestations of CD create a long differential diagnosis, which is shown in **Table 13-4**. On the other hand, the differential diagnosis for UC is limited to other causes of hematochezia and/or bloody diarrhea. The differential diagnosis for UC is summarized in **Table 13-5**.

TREATMENT

To date, no curative medical therapy exists for IBD. The goal of treatment is to achieve complete endoscopic and histologic remission, suppress symptoms,

Table 13-3. Findings of Inflammatory Bowel Disease on Physical Examination	
Category	**Findings**
Growth data	Height and weight velocity decreased for age, delayed puberty
General	Appear well or chronically ill
Abdomen	Tenderness, fullness, right lower quadrant mass
Genitourinary	Fistula
Rectal	Tags, tenderness, fissure, fistula, swelling, inflammation, stool guaiac
Extremities	Clubbing, arthritis
Dermatologic	Pallor, stomatitis, erythema nodosum, pyoderma gangrenosum

improve patients' quality of life, reduce the risk of recurrence, and avoid long-term complications, including intestinal perforation and strictures, to minimize the need for surgical procedures.

Medical Therapy

Multiple medications are effective in reducing symptoms, inducing remission, and preventing relapse. The intensity of treatment varies with the severity of disease. The pharmacologic agents used to treat IBD are divided into 5 categories: aminosalicylates, corticosteroids, antibiotics, immunomodulators, and biologics (**Table 13-6**). Traditionally, IBD has been treated in a stepwise approach, with more powerful agents reserved for patients whose condition does not improve with initial treatment. Patients with more severe disease at presentation are often treated with immunomodulators or biological agents soon after diagnosis. Aminosalicylates are effective for mild UC and Crohn's colitis, but are not effective in CD with small bowel involvement (Evidence Level II). Approximately 5% of patients have an allergic reaction to aminosalicylates, manifested as a rash and bloody diarrhea that can be difficult to distinguish from the symptoms of IBD. Systemic corticosteroids are effective in the initial treatment of moderate-to-severe IBD and are often the first choice to induce clinical remission (Evidence Level II-2). Prednisone does not reduce the risk of relapse and has

Box 13-1. Initial Evaluation of Children With Suspected Inflammatory Bowel Disease

Blood work
- CBC with differential
- Inflammatory markers (ESR, CRP)
- Liver function tests (ALT, alkaline phosphatase, bilirubin, GGT)
- Albumin
- Amylase and/or lipase

Stool studies
- *Salmonella, Shigella, Campylobacter, Yersinia*
- *Escherichia coli* O157
- *Clostridium difficile*
- Ova and parasites
- Lactoferrin or calprotectin
- Occult blood

Anticipatory management
- **Review immunization status**
  - Measles, mumps, and rubella
  - *Haemophilus influenzae*
  - Influenza
  - Pneumococcal
  - Inactivated polio vaccine
  - Varicella
  - Diphtheria, pertussis, acellular tetanus
  - Hepatitis A
  - Hepatitis B
  - Human papillomavirus
  - Meningitis
- **PPD skin test**

Abbreviations: ALT, alanine aminotransferase; CBC, complete blood cell count; CRP, C-reactive protein; ESR, erythrocyte sedimentation rate; GGT, γ-glutamyltransferase; PPD, purified protein derivative.

Reproduced with permission from Rufo PA, Denson LA, Sylvester FA, et al. Health supervision in the management of children and adolescents with IBD: NASPGHAN recommendations. *J Pediatr Gastroenterol Nutr.* 2012;55(1):93–108.

Table 13-4. Differential Diagnosis of Presenting Symptoms of Crohn Disease

Primary Presenting Symptom	Diagnostic Considerations
Right lower quadrant abdominal pain, with or without a mass	Appendicitis, infection (eg, *Campylobacter*, *Yersinia*), lymphoma, intussusception, mesenteric adenitis, Meckel diverticulum, ovarian cyst
Chronic periumbilical or epigastric abdominal pain	Irritable bowel, constipation, lactose intolerance, peptic disease, celiac disease
Rectal bleeding, no diarrhea	Fissure, polyp, Meckel diverticulum, rectal ulcer syndrome
Bloody diarrhea	Infection, hemolytic-uremic syndrome, Henoch-Schönlein purpura
Watery diarrhea	Irritable bowel, lactose intolerance, giardiasis, *Cryptosporidium*, sorbitol, laxatives
Perirectal disease	Fissure, hemorrhoid (rare), streptococcal infection, condyloma (rare)
Growth delay	Celiac disease, endocrinopathy
Anorexia, weight loss	Anorexia nervosa
Arthritis	Collagen vascular disease, infection
Liver abnormalities	Chronic hepatitis

Reproduced with permission from Wyllie R, Hyams JS, Kay M, eds. *Pediatric Gastrointestinal and Liver Disease*. 5th ed. Philadelphia, PA: Elsevier; 2016:511.

significant side effects with prolonged or repeated exposure; therefore, it should only be used for a limited time.

Immunomodulator therapy is frequently used for moderate IBD or for steroid-refractory or steroid-dependent disease. Thiopurines (azathioprine and 6-mercaptopurine) have been shown to decrease the risk of recurrence in patients in remission (Evidence Level II-1). Methotrexate is recommended primary maintenance therapy for patients with CD (Evidence Level II-3), but it is rarely used in patients with UC who fail to respond to thiopurines or do not tolerate thiopurines.

Table 13-5. Differential Diagnosis of Ulcerative Colitis in Children

Diagnostic Category	Specific Diagnosis
Enteric infection	*Salmonella, Shigella, Clostridium difficile, Campylobacter, Aeromonas, Yersinia,* enterohemorrhagic *Escherichia coli, Entamoeba histolytica, Giardia lamblia,*[a] cytomegalovirus,[b] norovirus
Pseudomembranous (post-antibiotic) enterocolitis	*Clostridium difficile*
Carbohydrate intolerance[a]	Lactose, sucrose, nondigestible carbohydrates (sorbitol, xylitol, mannitol, maltitol)
Vasculitis	Henoch-Schönlein purpura Hemolytic-uremic syndrome
Allergic enterocolitis[c]	—
Hirschsprung's enterocolitis[c]	—
Eosinophilic gastroenteritis	—
Celiac disease[a]	—
Laxative abuse[a]	—
Neoplasms	Juvenile polyp,[c] adenocarcinoma, intestinal polyposis
Immunodeficiencies	—

[a] Watery, nonbloody diarrhea.
[b] Primarily during flares of disease activity, especially in patients receiving immunomodulatory therapy.
[c] Primarily in the young child.

Modified from Park S-D, Markowitz JF. Ulcerative colitis (pediatric). In: Johnson L, ed. *Encyclopedia of Gastroenterology.* New York, NY: Academic Press; 2004:400–408, with permission.

The most widely used biologic therapies are the family of monoclonal antibodies to neutralize tumor necrosis factor (TNF). Over the past 20 years, infliximab has been of great benefit to many pediatric patients with CD by inducing and maintaining remission, allowing for mucosal healing, inducing perianal fistula closure, reducing corticosteroid exposure, promoting growth, and improving quality of life (Evidence Level II-1). Infliximab also has a role

Table 13-6. Medical Management of Inflammatory Bowel Disease

Treatment	Induction Maintenance	Common Adverse Effects	Monitoring
Aminosalicylates			
Sulfasalazine Balsalazide Mesalamine Olsalazine	Induction and maintenance	Nausea Anorexia Diarrhea Headache Nephritis	CBC, liver chemistries, BUN, and creatinine analysis
Antibiotics			
Metronidazole Ciprofloxacin	Induction	Nausea, glossitis, metallic taste, stomatitis, headache, urticaria, dry mouth, vaginal/ urethral burning Vaginal yeast infection	History and examination
Biologics			
Infliximab Adalimumab Certolizumab Golimumab Vedolizumab Ustekinumab Tofacitinib	Induction and maintenance	Nausea, fatigue, fever/ chills, hives, psoriatic rash, infusion/local reaction	PPD, chest radiograph, routine skin examination, CBC, liver chemistries
Corticosteroids	Induction	Growth disturbance, bone loss, hirsutism, hypertension, acne, hyperglycemia, facial swelling, weight gain, infection	Monitor growth, eye examination, PPD/ chest radiograph, bone density
Enteral nutrition	Induction and maintenance	Loose stools, nausea, nighttime waking	Check height and weight at each office visit

(continued)

Table 13-6. Medical Management of Inflammatory Bowel Disease (*continued*)

Treatment	Induction Maintenance	Common Adverse Effects	Monitoring
Immunomodulators			
6-MP Azathioprine Methotrexate	Induction and maintenance	Nausea, pancreatitis, vomiting, malaise, rash, fever, anorexia, stomatitis, hepatoxicity, marrow suppression	TPMT measurement, CBC, liver function tests, amylase, 6-MP metabolite levels
Immunosuppressants			
Cyclosporine Tacrolimus	Induction	Nausea, seizure, hepatitis, infection, nephrotoxicity, glucose intolerance	Pneumocystis, prophylaxis, chemistry panel, liver chemistries
		Hypertension	CBD, cholesterol, serum lipids, glucose

Abbreviations: BUN, blood urea nitrogen; CBC, complete blood cell count; 6-MP, 6-mercaptopurine; PPD, purified protein derivative (tuberculosis skin test); TPMT, thiopurine methyltransferase.

Reproduced with permission from Rufo PA, Denson LA, Sylvester FA, et al. Health supervision in the management of children and adolescents with IBD: NASPGHAN recommendations. *J Pediatr Gastroenterol Nutr.* 2012;55(1):93–108.

in the management of refractory pediatric UC, but overall its effectiveness is lower than that in pediatric CD. Adalimumab also is effective for pediatric CD (Evidence Level II-1), but its use in pediatric UC is reserved for patients who no longer respond to infliximab or do not tolerate infliximab (Evidence Level II-3). Other biologics (vedolizumab, ustekinumab, and tofacitinib) have been approved for adults with IBD, but pediatric data are limited. Unfortunately, the use of corticosteroids and immunomodulator and biologic therapies may not be without risks, such as opportunistic and serious infections, autoimmune diseases, and malignancies.

Patients with severe UC whose symptoms persist after 5 days of intravenous corticosteroid therapy require escalation to a second-line therapy (infliximab, tacrolimus, or cyclosporine) (Evidence Level II-3). Early consultation to pediatric surgery is advisable for possible colectomy if patient fails to respond to a second-line therapy (Evidence Level II-2).

Nutritional Therapy

Growth failure and malnutrition are common in patients with CD, and multiple factors are responsible for these symptoms. Enteral nutritional therapy with liquid formulas may be used in the management of pediatric CD. Exclusive enteral nutrition (EEN) can be effective in inducing remission in patients with newly diagnosed CD (Evidence Level I). On the other hand, partial enteral nutrition is not an effective induction therapy for CD (Evidence Level I). Exclusive enteral nutrition has been shown to promote mucosal healing, maintain longer-term remission, and enhance overall linear growth in patients with CD (Evidence Level II-3). Elemental, semielemental, and polymeric formulas have similar efficacy in inducing remission in pediatric CD (Evidence Level I). No clear benefit of total parenteral nutrition or EEN has been established for patients with severe UC (Evidence Level III).

Surgery

Surgery for IBD is reserved for very specific indications. Urgent surgical intervention is often needed for patients who develop a perforation or an abscess, or in cases of fulminant colitis. Surgery is often performed in children with CD who have localized disease of the small bowel or colon unresponsive to medical management, a bowel perforation, a stricture, and/or intractable intestinal bleeding. Whereas surgical options for CD are only palliative, colectomy for patients with UC is curative and should be performed for intractable disease, in cases of significant therapeutic complications, and in cases of fulminant disease that is unresponsive to medical therapy. The surgical treatment for UC is total colectomy with an ileal pouch-anal anastomosis. The most common long-term complication is pouchitis, which often responds to antibiotics (metronidazole or ciprofloxacin) (Evidence Level III). The probiotic VSL#3 is recommended for maintaining remission in patients with recurrent and/or chronic pouchitis (Evidence Level III).

LONG-TERM CONSIDERATIONS

The course of IBD is marked by remissions and exacerbations despite adherence to therapy. Crohn disease is associated with high morbidity but low mortality. Intestinal inflammation may recur despite treatment, often without any clinical symptoms. Therefore, close follow-up and surveillance laboratory tests, including fecal lactoferrin or calprotectin, are recommended (Evidence

Level II-2). The region of bowel involved and the complications of the inflammatory process (fistulas, strictures, and abscess formation) increase with time. Recent systematic reviews of the natural history of IBD in children have shown a reduction in the rates of surgery with the use of maintenance thiopurines and biologics (Evidence Level II-2). Unfortunately, many patients with CD require surgery; repeated resections may rarely lead to short bowel syndrome.

Most children with mild-to-moderate UC respond to the initial treatment, and many children with mild disease may remain in remission on a prophylactic aminosalicylate preparation. On the other hand, patients with severe or intractable UC require aggressive medical or surgical intervention. Overall, within 5 years of diagnosis, approximately 20% of patients with UC will undergo a colectomy. The risk of colon cancer increases rapidly after 10 years with the disease; therefore, surveillance colonoscopies should be performed after 8 years of disease.

SUGGESTED READING

Critch J, Day AS, Otley A, King-Moore C, Teitelbaum JE, Shashidhar H; NASPGHAN IBD Committee. Use of enteral nutrition for the control of intestinal inflammation in pediatric Crohn disease. *J Pediatr Gastroenterol Nutr*. 2012;54(2):298–305

de Bie CI, Escher JC, de Ridder L. Antitumor necrosis factor treatment for pediatric inflammatory bowel disease. *Inflamm Bowel Dis*. 2012;18(5):985–1002

Pappa H, Thayu M, Sylvester F, Leonard M, Zemel B, Gordon C. Skeletal health of children and adolescents with inflammatory bowel disease. *J Pediatr Gastroenterol Nutr*. 2011;53(1):11–25

Ruemmele FM, Veres G, Kolho KL, et al; European Crohn's and Colitis Organisation; European Society of Pediatric Gastroenterology, Hepatology and Nutrition. Consensus guidelines of ECCO/ESPGHAN on the medical management of pediatric Crohn's disease. *J Crohns Colitis*. 2014;8(10):1179–1207

Rufo PA, Denson LA, Sylvester FA, et al. Health supervision in the management of children and adolescents with IBD: NASPGHAN recommendations. *J Pediatr Gastroenterol Nutr*. 2012;55(1):93–108

Turner D, Ruemmele FM, Orlanski-Meyer E, et al. Management of paediatric ulcerative colitis, part 1: ambulatory care—an evidence-based guideline from European Crohn's and Colitis Organization and European Society of Paediatric Gastroenterology, Hepatology, and Nutrition. *J Pediatr Gastroenterol Nutr*. 2018:67(2):257–291

Jaundice and Liver Disease

Ryan T. Fischer, MD, and James F. Daniel, MD

OVERVIEW AND DEFINITIONS

Jaundice is an uncommon but potentially serious finding in children that reflects significant hyperbilirubinemia. For jaundice to be detected, the serum bilirubin level is usually greater than 2 to 3 mg/dL; some children with elevated bilirubin levels related to significant conditions do not have visible jaundice. Hyperbilirubinemia and jaundice in infants, especially within the first 2 weeks after birth, are typically physiologic but may be a harbinger of underlying disease.

Elevated bilirubin levels may be mainly unconjugated or conjugated. Many causes of unconjugated hyperbilirubinemia are not associated with liver damage but represent the defective metabolism or overproduction of unconjugated bilirubin. However, conjugated hyperbilirubinemia is often associated with intrinsic or extrinsic liver disease and the retention of bile in the liver, which is usually termed *cholestasis*. On occasion, cholestasis can be self-limited and/or related to a nonspecific infection, but it might be indicative of more serious conditions that can require long-term treatment or liver transplantation or lead to death.

Bilirubin Metabolism

Understanding the causes of hyperbilirubinemia and cholestasis in children requires a basic understanding of bilirubin metabolism. Bilirubin is a pigmented waste product primarily produced from the breakdown of heme, a component of hemoglobin found in red blood cells. When heme is released from hemoglobin, it is converted to biliverdin and then to bilirubin, which is in its unconjugated form. In the liver, unconjugated bilirubin is conjugated with glucuronic acid, making it water soluble and capable of being excreted in the bile.

Most laboratory assays measure total bilirubin levels in milligrams per deciliter. In a jaundiced child, as well as in a child with an elevated serum bilirubin level without jaundice, the bilirubin should always be fractionated. Doing so allows for assessment of whether the patient's hyperbilirubinemia is mostly conjugated (estimated by measurement of the direct—or water-soluble—form of bilirubin) or unconjugated (reported by laboratories as *indirect bilirubin,* which is calculated by subtracting the direct bilirubin measurement from the total). Significant indirect (unconjugated) hyperbilirubinemia leads to a differential diagnosis that is much different from that for direct (conjugated) or mixed hyperbilirubinemia. Although the terms *indirect* and *direct* bilirubin are often used for unconjugated and conjugated bilirubin, they are not completely equivalent. Measurement of direct bilirubin levels often overestimates the actual amount of conjugated bilirubin present for a variety of reasons. For simplicity, only the terms *unconjugated* and *conjugated* bilirubin will be used hereafter.

Unconjugated hyperbilirubinemia is usually attributable to the increased production or disordered metabolism of unconjugated bilirubin. Increased production of bilirubin is typical in most hemolytic anemias and hemoglobinopathies. Heritable conditions such as Gilbert syndrome and Crigler-Najjar syndrome are characterized by the reduced or absent conjugation of bilirubin. Conjugated hyperbilirubinemia is often the result of hepatocellular dysfunction or obstruction, which leads to cholestasis and the retention of bile. However, some heritable conditions are associated with a conjugated hyperbilirubinemia *without* cholestasis. Familiarity with the differential diagnosis for both unconjugated and conjugated hyperbilirubinemia is important in defining the best approach to managing a child with jaundice.

CAUSES AND DIFFERENTIAL DIAGNOSIS

The more commonly encountered diagnoses are presented in **Table 14-1.**

CLINICAL FEATURES OF HYPERBILIRUBINEMIA IN CHILDREN AND ADOLESCENTS

Unconjugated Hyperbilirubinemia

The most common causes of unconjugated hyperbilirubinemia that affect infants include physiologic jaundice of the newborn, human milk jaundice, ABO or Rh incompatibility, hemoglobinopathies, and red cell enzyme defects. **Table 14-1** lists the most common causes of unconjugated hyperbilirubinemia in older children, which are broadly separated into those associated with hemolysis (and the increased production of unconjugated bilirubin) and those associated with the decreased ability to conjugate unconjugated bilirubin. However, some

continued on page 163

Table 14-1. Clinical Clues and Additional Workup to Aid in Diagnosing the Older Child or Adolescent With Jaundice

Category	Specific Disease	Clinical Signs and Symptoms	Helpful Diagnostic Examinations
Primarily Unconjugated Hyperbilirubinemia			
Hemolysis			
Inherited and acquired hemolytic conditions are associated with high indirect bilirubin, anemia, reticulocytosis, elevated lactate dehydrogenase, decreased haptoglobin, and possible pathognomonic findings on peripheral smear.	Sickle cell anemia	Vaso-occlusive (pain) crises, splenic sequestration	Newborn screen, hemoglobin electrophoresis
	Spherocytosis	Splenomegaly, milder anemia	Peripheral smear, osmotic fragility test
	Thalassemia	Asymptomatic to transfusion dependent (spectrum)	Newborn screen, hemoglobin electrophoresis
	G6PD deficiency	X-linked, acute anemia after exposure to oxidative chemicals, stress	G6PD enzyme activity
	Autoimmune hemolytic anemia	Anemia, splenomegaly	Direct antiglobulin test (Coombs)
	Malaria	Paroxysms of fevers, shaking chills	Thick and thin peripheral smear, immunochromatographic testing, PCR

(continued)

Table 14-1. Clinical Clues and Additional Workup to Aid in Diagnosing the Older Child or Adolescent With Jaundice (*continued*)

Category	Specific Disease	Clinical Signs and Symptoms	Helpful Diagnostic Examinations
Primarily Unconjugated Hyperbilirubinemia (*continued*)			
Inherited Unconjugated Hyperbilirubinemias			
These disorders are due to an inherited inability to conjugate bilirubin. Mutations in the uridine-glucuronosyltransferase *UGT1A1* gene prevent adequate or any conjugation of bilirubin. Gilbert syndrome typically presents with a mild elevation of indirect bilirubin levels without evidence of hemolysis or liver disease. Without prompt treatment, Crigler-Najjar types I and II can be associated with severe indirect hyperbilirubinemia and kernicterus (especially type I).	Gilbert syndrome	Asymptomatic, recurrent jaundice	No specific testing indicated
	Crigler-Najjar syndrome (I and II)	Persistent, moderate-to-severe jaundice, kernicterus (type I)	Response to phenobarbital (type II), measured transferase activity, genetic testing
Primarily Conjugated or Mixed Hyperbilirubinemia			
Obstructive			
Obstructions often associated with elevations in GGT and alkaline phosphatase, indicators of stress on cholangiocytes of bile ducts. Elevations in transaminases may not be as prominent.	Gallstones	Colicky, right upper quadrant abdominal pain, nausea, vomiting, fevers; more common in females and adolescents or those with exposure to parenteral nutrition	Imaging of right upper quadrant with ultrasound or MRCP

Table 14-1. Clinical Clues and Additional Workup to Aid in Diagnosing the Older Child or Adolescent With Jaundice (continued)

Category	Specific Disease	Clinical Signs and Symptoms	Helpful Diagnostic Examinations
Primarily Conjugated or Mixed Hyperbilirubinemia (continued)			
Obstructive (continued)	Tumor	Hepatomegaly, constitutional systems	Imaging of liver, α-fetoprotein level, biopsy
	Parasite (ascaris, schistosomiasis)	Travel to endemic areas, abdominal pain, fever, hepatosplenomegaly	Stool ova and parasite examination, antigen testing
Infectious	Sepsis	Abnormal body temperature, tachycardia, respiratory distress, hypotension, mental status changes	Blood, urine, spinal fluid culture
Clinical findings of sepsis should be dealt with promptly; sepsis should always be considered in infants with jaundice. Many infections can cause liver inflammation, but hepatitis A, B, C, D, E are primarily hepatotropic. Acute presentations of viral hepatitis can include fulminant hepatic failure.	Hepatitis A, B, C, and others	Fever, malaise, nausea, vomiting	Hepatitis A IgM; hepatitis B core IgM, hepatitis B surface antigen; hepatitis C IgG; serologic or PCR testing for other viruses (ie, Epstein-Barr, cytomegalovirus, HIV) as indicated; liver biopsy

(continued)

Table 14-1. Clinical Clues and Additional Workup to Aid in Diagnosing the Older Child or Adolescent With Jaundice (*continued*)

Category	Specific Disease	Clinical Signs and Symptoms	Helpful Diagnostic Examinations
Primarily Conjugated or Mixed Hyperbilirubinemia (*continued*)			
Drugs and Toxins			
Clues to drug-induced liver disease include timing of exposures and amount of drug ingested. Acute injuries often associated with significant elevations in AST and ALT. Acetaminophen toxicity may also result from chronic inadvertent overdoses. Reactions to any drug may be idiosyncratic and unrelated to dose.	Acetaminophen	Mental status changes, encephalopathy, nausea, vomiting	Acetaminophen level; screening for drugs of abuse
	Mushroom poisoning	Appropriate exposure history, gastrointestinal symptoms, encephalopathy, renal insufficiency	No direct laboratory measurement; screening for other drug ingestions can be useful.
Autoimmune Liver Disease			
Autoimmune disease tends to present in adolescence, perhaps due to the influence of hormones. Fulminant presentations associated with failure are rare. Steroid therapy and long-term immunosuppression are mainstays for autoimmune hepatitis. Sclerosing cholangitis therapy is mostly supportive, as immunosuppressive therapies are ineffective.	AIH	Arthritis, colitis, erythema nodosum, other autoimmune diseases. Drug-induced AIH is associated with minocycline.	Antinuclear antibody, quantitative IgG, anti–smooth muscle antibody, anti–liver-kidney microsomal antibody
	Primary sclerosing cholangitis	80%–90% of patients have or will develop colitis.	p-ANCA, MRCP, screening endoscopy, "onion skinning" on liver biopsy

Table 14-1. Clinical Clues and Additional Workup to Aid in Diagnosing the Older Child or Adolescent With Jaundice (*continued*)

Category	Specific Disease	Clinical Signs and Symptoms	Helpful Diagnostic Examinations
Primarily Conjugated or Mixed Hyperbilirubinemia (*continued*)			
Autoimmune Liver Disease			
	Celiac disease	Diarrhea, malabsorption, abdominal pain, gluten intolerance	Tissue transglutaminase antibodies (IgA or IgG), antiendomysial antibodies
Metabolic and Genetic Disorders			
A variety of inherited diseases. Management is generally lifelong, with careful attention to disease progression and the potential for (curative) transplantation.	Wilson disease	Kayser-Fleischer rings, hemolysis, neuropsychiatric findings, Fanconi syndrome	Low ceruloplasmin (<20 mg/dL), elevated 24-hour urine copper (>100 mcg/d), hepatic copper content on biopsy >50–250 mcg/g dry weight; mutation in *ATP7B* gene
	α_1-antitrypsin deficiency	Hepatomegaly associated with pulmonary disease in older patients	α_1-antitrypsin phenotype (PiZZ associated with liver disease), low α_1-antitrypsin serum levels, periodic acid Schiff staining of liver biopsy specimen reveals diastase-resistant hepatocyte inclusions.

(continued)

Table 14-1. Clinical Clues and Additional Workup to Aid in Diagnosing the Older Child or Adolescent With Jaundice (*continued*)

Category	Specific Disease	Clinical Signs and Symptoms	Helpful Diagnostic Examinations
Primarily Conjugated or Mixed Hyperbilirubinemia (*continued*)			
Metabolic and Genetic Disorders (continued)			
	Hemochromatosis	Rare presentation in children, associated with bronze diabetes, arthropathy	Elevated serum ferritin and transferrin saturation, elevated hepatic iron content on biopsy, *HFE* gene testing
	Primary familial intrahepatic cholestasis	Intense pruritis, growth failure, hepatomegaly	Cholestasis in PFIC 1 and 2 associated with low or normal GGT; PFIC 3 associated with high GGT; electron microscopy of liver biopsy specimen can reveal changes in bile appearance; specific gene testing can be diagnostic.
	Cystic fibrosis	Pulmonary disease, growth failure, hepatomegaly	Sweat chloride; *CFTR* gene testing
	Nonalcoholic fatty liver disease	Obesity, insulin resistance, hypertension, dyslipidemia	Steatosis noted on imaging; liver biopsy demonstrating >5% macrovesicular steatosis, ballooning hepatocellular injury, and possibly fibrosis

Table 14-1. Clinical Clues and Additional Workup to Aid in Diagnosing the Older Child or Adolescent With Jaundice (continued)

Category	Specific Disease	Clinical Signs and Symptoms	Helpful Diagnostic Examinations
Primarily Conjugated or Mixed Hyperbilirubinemia (continued)			
Vascular Anomalies			
Rare in children with no risk factors. Potential risks include family history of thrombosis, exposure to certain medications, and receipt of myeloablative chemotherapy in the setting of stem cell transplantation.	Budd-Chiari syndrome	Abdominal pain (occasionally acute), ascites, hepatomegaly, history of oral contraceptives	Doppler ultrasonography, angiography
	Veno-occlusive disease	Abdominal pain, hepatomegaly, ascites, history of chemotherapy	Doppler ultrasonography, liver biopsy
Disorders of Intrahepatic Ducts			
These disorders include conditions associated with a paucity of bile ducts (eg, Alagille syndrome) and fibrocystic condition associated with bile duct disarray. These conditions often are inherited and associated with systemic disease.	Alagille syndrome	Triangular facies with wide forehead, prominent chin; peripheral pulmonic stenosis, butterfly vertebrae, renal dysplasia, poor linear growth	Liver biopsy demonstrating a paucity of bile ducts; hypercholesterolemia (>200 mg/dL); hypertriglyceridemia (>500 mg/dL); genetic testing for JAG1 mutations
	Congenital hepatic fibrosis	Hepatomegaly, portal hypertension, polycystic kidney disease, recurrent cholangitis	Diagnosis established by abdominal ultrasonography, MRCP; liver biopsy can be useful.

(continued)

Table 14-1. Clinical Clues and Additional Workup to Aid in Diagnosing the Older Child or Adolescent With Jaundice (*continued*)

Category	Specific Disease	Clinical Signs and Symptoms	Helpful Diagnostic Examinations
Primarily Conjugated or Mixed Hyperbilirubinemia (*continued*)			
Inherited Conjugated Hyperbilirubinemia			
Direct hyperbilirubinemia without evidence of liver disease or cholestasis, likely due to an inherited disorder of conjugated bilirubin metabolism. While the jaundice can be concerning from a nonmedical perspective, there is no need for treatment or longitudinal testing.	Dubin-Johnson syndrome	Asymptomatic	Urine coproporphyrin fractions; total coproporphyrin is normal, but coproporphyrin I fraction is 3–4 times higher than III (inversion of normal ratio); black liver on autopsy.
	Rotor syndrome	Asymptomatic	High total coproporphyrin; coproporphyrin I fraction not as dominant as in Dubin-Johnson syndrome

Abbreviations: AIH, autoimmune hepatitis; ALT, alanine aminotransferase; AST, aspartate aminotransferase; GGT, γ-glutamyltransferase; G6PD, glucose-6-phosphate dehydrogenase; MRCP: magnetic resonance cholangiopancreatography; p-ANCA, peripheral antinuclear cytoplasmic antibody; PCR, polymerase chain reaction; PFIC, progressive familial intrahepatic cholestasis.

causes, such as the hyperbilirubinemia seen with sepsis, disseminated intra-vascular coagulation, hematomas, and polycythemia, do not fit easily into the unconjugated or conjugated hyperbilirubinemia categories.

Gilbert Syndrome

Gilbert syndrome is associated with mild, recurrent elevations in unconjugated bilirubin with otherwise normal liver enzyme levels. Often, these bilirubin elevations are noted at times of illness or stress. The disorder is benign, and management consists of reassurance. However, if bilirubin levels are regularly greater than 5 mg/dL, the clinician should consider an evaluation for hemolytic disease or genetic testing of the *UGT1A1* gene to rule out Crigler-Najjar syndrome.

Crigler-Najjar Syndrome

This disorder usually presents with jaundice at birth or in early infancy. Unconjugated hyperbilirubinemia can be severe enough to lead to kernicterus, central nervous system injury caused by the accumulation of unconjugated bilirubin. Crigler-Najjar syndrome is divided into 2 types. Type 1 (CN1) is very severe; affected individuals often die in childhood as a result of kernicterus. However, with proper treatment, they may survive longer. Type 2 (CN2) is less severe, and patients are less likely to develop kernicterus. Most affected individuals survive into adulthood. Crigler-Najjar syndrome is caused by mutations in the *UGT1A1* gene (controlling production of the bilirubin uridine diphosphate glucuronosyltransferase [UGT] enzyme), which is found primarily in liver cells and is necessary for the removal of bilirubin from the body. Individuals with CN1 have no enzyme function, whereas those with CN2 have less than 20% normal function. The loss of bilirubin-UGT function decreases glucuronidation of unconjugated bilirubin, leading to unconjugated hyperbilirubinemia, jaundice, and often kernicterus.

Conjugated Hyperbilirubinemia

Table 14-1 lists some of the causes of conjugated hyperbilirubinemia in older children, which can be grouped into those associated with obstruction of the extrahepatic biliary tree (eg, gallstones, anatomic abnormalities, tumor, parasites) and those associated with intrinsic forms of liver disease. Intrinsic forms of disease can include infectious, autoimmune, metabolic, and genetic conditions. While severe intrinsic disease is rare, these conditions pose a risk of progression to significant fibrosis or cirrhosis of the liver, and a possible need for transplantation.

Gallstones

Cholelithiasis (the presence of solid concretions or stones in the gallbladder) is uncommon in healthy children, occurring mainly in girls and during puberty. Risk factors include obesity, hemolytic disease, and a history of parenteral nutrition. Cholelithiasis alone may not cause a significant elevation in the bilirubin or liver enzymes. However, if the gallstone or gallstones migrate from the gallbladder into the biliary tree, they can become lodged and result in an obstructive cholestasis, often punctuated by colicky biliary pain and inflammation or infection of the gallbladder and/or liver. Hyperbilirubinemia associated with an obstructive gallstone is typically conjugated, but unconjugated hyperbilirubinemia may be seen if the stones are secondary to chronic hemolysis. Transaminase levels may be significantly elevated, but γ-glutamyltransferase (GGT) and alkaline phosphatase elevations are typical when the bilirubin level is abnormal as a result of obstruction. Diagnosis is best achieved by ultrasonography followed by magnetic resonance imaging (specifically, magnetic resonance cholangiopancreatography [MRCP]) if there is the possibility of a stone in the common bile duct (choledocholithiasis). Management includes endoscopic retrograde cholangiopancreatography (ERCP) with stone extraction and/or sphincterotomy if there is choledocholithiasis, followed by or concomitant with cholecystectomy.

Drug Injury

Drug-induced liver injury (DILI) is a rare but potentially serious cause of conjugated hyperbilirubinemia and cholestasis in children. A recent report from the DILI Network implicated minocycline (associated with an autoimmune hepatitis-like scenario), isoniazid, amoxicillin, azithromycin, atomoxetine, and lamotrigine as the most common agents in children with suspected DILI. Almost any drug can cause DILI; jaundice, in particular, in DILI has a poor prognosis. Steroids for sports performance and drugs for weight loss are some of the most common causes of DILI, and children are at high risk. Acetaminophen overdose, often intentional in teenagers, is another potentially serious cause of DILI.

Autoimmune Liver Disease

Primary sclerosing cholangitis (PSC) and autoimmune hepatitis (AIH) are 2 of the more common causes of hyperbilirubinemia/jaundice with cholestasis in older children. Certain risk factors, including certain drugs (eg, minocycline for AIH) and other autoimmune diseases (ulcerative colitis for PSC, Crohn disease for AIH) can put a child at risk of developing 1 of these autoimmune liver diseases, which are idiopathic in most affected children. Autoimmune hepatitis is more common in girls and sometimes is seen in children with other autoimmune disorders. The disease is diagnosed by means of liver histology (interface hepatitis, plasma cell infiltrates) and laboratory tests that demonstrate elevated levels of several autoantibodies and IgG. Antinuclear antibodies, anti-smooth muscle or anti-F-actin antibodies, and/or anti–liver-kidney microsomal antibodies may be elevated in AIH. Primary sclerosing cholangitis has pathognomonic histology (portal fibrosis, "onion skinning") and can be associated with peripheral antinuclear cytoplasmic antibody positivity. However, the histologic findings can be subject to sampling error, and the diagnosis typically is made based on a "beaded" appearance of the biliary tree on MRCP. Treatment for AIH consists of a steroid-based immunosuppressive regimen in combination with long-term immunosuppression with azathioprine (Evidence Level I). Treatment for PSC is mostly supportive, with use of ursodiol for choleresis (Evidence Level I); investigations into other therapeutics (eg, vancomycin) are also underway.

Hepatitis A, B, and C
See Chapter 10.

Wilson Disease
In children with Wilson disease, copper metabolism is disordered from birth, but the clinical presentation almost always occurs after 5 years of age. Associated signs of Wilson disease can include a mixed hyperbilirubinemia with relatively mild elevations in transaminases, Coomb-negative hemolysis, and Fanconi syndrome (renal tubular wasting). Diagnosis is based on a low serum ceruloplasmin level, an elevated urine copper level in a 24-hour collection, histologic findings, and (more commonly now) genetic testing. Treatment should be instituted quickly after diagnosis and includes a low copper diet, chelation therapy with penicillamine or trientene to bind copper and excrete it in the urine, and zinc to abrogate copper absorption in the intestine (Evidence Level I). Zinc may be used as a preventive measure in presymptomatic Wilson disease (eg, discovered in a sibling of an affected patient), but there is concern regarding treatment failure with zinc monotherapy.

Elevated Transaminases Without Jaundice
An increasingly common challenge for those who care for children and adolescents is evaluating and managing isolated elevated transaminases. These patients are usually asymptomatic, and the condition is sometimes detected as an incidental finding when general laboratory studies are obtained. These findings may include elevations of both alanine aminotransferase (ALT) and aspartate aminotransferase (AST) without elevations of bilirubin, GGT, or alkaline phosphatase. What is remarkable is the absence of cholestasis in these

children. The causes of isolated elevated transaminase levels are broad and
include nonalcoholic fatty liver disease (NAFLD)/nonalcoholic steatohepatitis
(NASH), infection (hepatitis A, B, and C; other viral and parasitic infections),
celiac disease, thyroid disease, iron overload, neuromuscular disease, and
medication or supplement use. Detection of patients with elevated transaminases in the absence of jaundice has become more common in the past few years
as a result of the worldwide obesity epidemic and its associated incidence of
NAFLD/NASH. Of note, ALT may be the only abnormal laboratory value in up
to 20% of these children; in contrast to alcohol injury, however, the AST-ALT
ratio in NAFLD is usually less than 1.0. The pathogenesis of NAFLD/NASH is
multifactorial and related to overwhelming the liver's capacity to handle primary
metabolic energy substrates (carbohydrates and fatty acids), leading to accumulation of toxic lipid species. This accumulation induces hepatocellular stress,
injury, and death, leading to fibrosis and genomic instability that predispose
the patient to cirrhosis and hepatocellular carcinoma. Fatty acids appear to be
essential modifiers in the development of NASH, and genetic predisposition
appears to be another important consideration in many affected individuals.

EVALUATION

Crucial factors are the timing of the detection of hyperbilirubinemia and
whether the patient has had any fevers, abdominal pain, anorexia, nausea,
vomiting, fatigue, pruritis, darkening of the urine, easy bruising or bleeding
(eg, nosebleeds or bleeding from the gums while brushing), or any other
concerning symptoms. Excessive weight gain may be due to ascites. Pale
or clay-colored stools may indicate obstructive liver disease or more severe
hepatic injury. Melena or hematochezia may be due to variceal bleeding
associated with portal hypertension.

Few pediatricians or primary care physicians will diagnose or manage many
of these conditions; however, they will partner with a gastroenterologist in caring
for these children. The primary care physician can be most effective in responding promptly to signs of jaundice and/or hyperbilirubinemia (eg, recognizing
the need to immediately change the care of a newborn with conjugated bilirubin
[evaluating for sepsis, discontinuing lactose and fructose/sucrose, testing of
thyroid hormone, international normalized ratio]).

If hyperbilirubinemia is detected, the physical examination should include
characterization of any signs of jaundice; an assessment of the abdomen for
tenderness, ascites, hepatomegaly, splenomegaly, or mass; and careful evaluation for the stigmata of liver disease, including palmar erythema, gynecomastia
in boys, caput medusae, and spider angioma. Liver failure can be associated

with encephalopathy; therefore, assessing for neurologic changes (sleepiness, confusion, decreased activity, tremor) is necessary. Cholestasis may present with xanthomas, especially in patients with Alagille syndrome and familial cholestasis. Cholestasis also may result in micronutrient deficiencies, leading to night blindness and xerophthalmia (vitamin A), rickets (vitamin D), tremor and loss of vibratory sense and proprioception (vitamin E), and easy bleeding from the nose or gums (vitamin K). A rash that is or resembles acrodermatitis enteropathica can be due to zinc or essential fatty acid deficiency. **Box 14-1** shows routine laboratory studies for the child with jaundice.

In a child or an adolescent with isolated, asymptomatic, elevated transaminases, the first priority is to repeat the tests to confirm the results. No consensus exists regarding appropriate timing for retesting, but the laboratory tests are usually repeated within a few weeks. Because of the wide range of normal results for alkaline phosphatase in children, obtaining a GGT can help determine whether there is any significant cholestatic involvement. In many asymptomatic children, abnormal values can revert to normal when the test is redone. Up to 70% of patients with isolated elevated transaminases will experience normalization within 6 months. In addition, a fluctuating pattern (transient/self-limiting or intermittent) is sometimes observed, and the test may need to be repeated more than once, even for a mild increase in transaminase levels. In areas with a high prevalence of hepatitis B virus (HBV) and hepatitis C virus (HCV) infection and in high-risk populations, clinicians should obtain viral markers at the time of repeated testing to accelerate the screening protocol. Some investigators recommend that HBV and HCV screening be pursued in all asymptomatic patients with mild transaminase elevations. Children with persistent and/or worsening isolated elevated liver enzyme levels should undergo further evaluation similar to that in children with conjugated hyperbilirubinemia (see **Box 14-1**). The gold standard for diagnosing NAFLD/NASH is identifying fat-laden hepatocytes or portal inflammation on biopsy; however, biopsy is generally reserved for cases in which the diagnosis remains uncertain.

MANAGEMENT

Hyperbilirubinemia and jaundice in the setting of sepsis, encephalopathy, or vitamin K–nonresponsive coagulopathy is a medical emergency best handled at an experienced, tertiary care center. Moreover, it is reasonable to refer any child with conjugated hyperbilirubinemia without a clear surgical cause to a pediatric gastroenterologist for accurate diagnosis and management.

Basic treatments for children with cholestatic liver disease are presented in **Table 14-2**.

Box 14-1. Useful Laboratory and Radiographic Investigations for the Older Child or Adolescent With Conjugated Hyperbilirubinemia

Initial screening
- Laboratory testing
  - Complete blood cell count with differential
  - Basic metabolic panel
  - Liver enzymes: alanine aminotransferase, aspartate aminotransferase, γ-glutamyltransferase, alkaline phosphatase
  - Fractionated bilirubin
  - Prothrombin time, international normalized ratio

Secondary screening (if cholestasis present)
- Abdominal ultrasonography (with Doppler, if indicated)
- Laboratory testing
  - Hepatitis A, B, and C serologies
  - Antinuclear antibody, quantitative IgG, anti-smooth muscle antibody, anti–liver-kidney microsomal antibody
  - Perinuclear antineutrophil cytoplasmic antibodies
  - Ferritin, transferrin saturation, iron, total iron-binding capacity
  - α_1-antitrypsin phenotype
  - Ceruloplasmin, 24-hour urine copper collection
  - Tissue transglutaminase IgA, quantitative IgA level
  - α-fetoprotein
  - Lactate, pyruvate, ammonia
  - Serum amino acids, urine organic acids, acylcarnitine profile
  - Specific gene mutation testing when indicated/available

Table 14-2. Medical Therapy for Children With Chronic Cholestasis (Evidence Level II-1 to II-3)

Therapeutic Category	Treatment	Dosage	Toxicity
Vitamin deficiency	Vitamin A	1,000–10,000 IU/d	Hepatotoxicity, central nervous system disease, bone and muscle pain; toxicity with >25,000 IU/d
	Vitamin D	400–1,000 IU/d	Hypercalcuria, hypercalcemia, gastrointestinal complaints (rare); toxicity with 40,000 IU/d
	Vitamin E	100–1,000 IU/d	Bleeding, coagulopathy; doses >1,600 IU/d
	Vitamin K	1–25 mg/d	No known toxicity; allergic reactions possible
Malabsorption	Medium-chain triglycerides	5–45 mL/d	Gastrointestinal complaints
	Long-chain triglycerides (corn, safflower oil, oral lipid emulsions)	Based on dietary needs	Gastrointestinal complaints
Pruritis	Cholestyramine	240 mg/kg/d divided 2–3 times/d	Fat-soluble vitamin deficiency, constipation, decreased absorption of other drugs
	Hydroxyzine	50–100 mg/d divided twice daily	Drowsiness, dizziness
	Rifampin	10–20 mg/kg/d once daily	Hepatotoxicity, bone marrow suppression, flu-like symptoms
Cholestasis (and pruritis)	Ursodiol	15–20 mg/kg/d divided twice daily	Diarrhea, increased pruritis

In unconjugated hyperbilirubinemia, patients require care directed toward treating the underlying disorder. In Gilbert syndrome, the disease course is benign, and no medication is required. Crigler-Najjar syndrome (types I and II) causes severe unconjugated hyperbilirubinemia, and patients benefit from phototherapy and, in the case of type II, enzyme induction with phenobarbital.

Conjugated hyperbilirubinemias associated with cholestasis can be treated with certain choleretic agents such as ursodeoxycholic acid (see **Table 14-2**). Ursodeoxycholic acid protects hepatocytes as a more water-soluble bile acid, capable of solubilizing cholesterol and reducing bile viscosity while competitively inhibiting the absorption of hydrophobic (and more toxic) endogenous bile acids. Another agent, the barbiturate phenobarbital, induces cytochrome P450–regulated bile excretion and has been used to treat cholestasis in some patients. However, use of phenobarbital for this purpose remains controversial, and phenobarbital treatment for choleresis is not recommended.

Antipruritic medications including antihistamines, ursodeoxycholic acid, and bile salt–binding agents such as cholestyramine may be used in moderate-to-severe cases, but their efficacy is limited. Instead, rifampin may be useful in selected patients.

More invasive interventions often are necessary to manage obstructive cholestasis, such as ERCP with distal bile duct stone extraction, sphincterotomy of the ampulla, or stent placement. In many cases, ERCP should be followed by or concomitant with cholecystectomy or other definitive surgery to address the underlying cause of biliary tree obstruction. Ursodiol has been used for stone dissolution, with limited efficacy.

In children or adolescents with isolated elevated transaminases, the evaluation will drive the management. For children being treated with any of the many medications associated with elevated transaminases, discontinuation of the potentially hepatotoxic medication and monitoring to determine a beneficial response to medication withdrawal is important. Treatment of a related systemic disorder is often associated with improvement in the liver enzyme levels. The primary treatment for NAFLD consists of behavioral modification, including weight loss, exercise, and adherence to a low-fat diet, in addition to tight glycemic control and correction of any underlying lipid abnormalities. Studies have demonstrated that a 7% to 10% reduction in body weight is associated with decreased inflammation in NAFLD, although no strict guidelines have been established. Given the prevalence of NAFLD and the need for longitudinal treatment, primary care physicians can play an important role in long-term monitoring and management of patients with fatty liver disease.

▼△▼△▼△▼△▼△▼△▼△▼△   ▽△▼△▼△▼△▼△▼△▼△▼△▼

LONG-TERM MONITORING

The longitudinal assessment of the growth and development of a child with cholestasis and chronic liver disease is crucial. Because of malabsorption and increased caloric and nutritional requirements, these children may not achieve typical expected growth. In advanced liver disease, ascites may develop, and the weight of retained fluid may convince a physician that growth is steady when, in reality, the patient may be losing lean muscle mass.

Caloric goals generally include 125% of recommended daily allowances based on weight for height at the 50th percentile. Recommended daily allowances of protein for age (2–3 g/kg/d in infants, 1–2 g/kg/d in older children) need to be followed. Protein restriction in encephalopathic patients is not recommended (Evidence Level I).

Supplementation with medium-chain triglycerides that are easily absorbed in the duodenum is recommended as a good source of fat calories. Essential fatty acid deficiency (manifest by an acrodermatitis enteropathica-like rash, growth impairment, and thrombocytopenia) can occur in patients with chronic liver disease. Evaluating the triene-to-tetraene ratio, which should be less than 0.3, can aid in diagnosis. Supplementation of long-chain fatty acids, usually with oral lipid emulsions, is effective (Evidence Level II-2).

Because of fat malabsorption, fat-soluble vitamin (A, D, E, and K) deficiency is common in cholestatic children. Symptoms can include xerophthalmia and night blindness (vitamin A), rickets (vitamin D), ataxia, loss of proprioception and vibratory sensation (vitamin E), and easy bleeding from gums or nosebleeds (vitamin K). Super-therapeutic doses of water-soluble forms of these vitamins are generally administered in cholestatic children. Serum levels of vitamins A, D, and E should be checked regularly. Measurement of vitamin K is useless, as it reflects only the most recent ingestion of K; therefore, the international normalized ratio of the prothrombin time, while not perfect, is measured as a function of vitamin K sufficiency.

Immunizations in all children, especially those with chronic liver disease, should be up-to-date; vaccines include both hepatitis A and B and any live vaccines that may be contraindicated after liver transplantation.

Finally, children with chronic liver disease are at risk of developing hepatocellular carcinoma in the setting of hepatic inflammation, fibrosis, or cirrhosis. A screening ultrasound every 6 months is recommended in these situations for adults with chronic liver disease (Evidence Level II-2). This recommendation may apply to children as well, and many liver programs monitor children with ultrasonography and check alpha-fetoprotein (a tumor marker) levels on a regular basis.

SUGGESTED READING

Brumbaugh D, Mack C. Conjugated hyperbilirubinemia in children. *Pediatr Rev*. 2012;33(7): 291–302

D'Agata ID, Balistreri WF. Evaluation of liver disease in the pediatric patient. *Pediatr Rev*. 1999; 20(11):376–390

El-Shabrawi MH, Kamal NM. Medical management of chronic liver diseases (CLD) in children (part II): focus on the complications of CLD, and CLD that require special considerations. *Pediatr Drugs*. 2011;13(6):371–383

Feranchak AP, Suchy FJ, Sokol RJ. Medical and nutritional management of cholestasis in infants and children. In: Suchy FJ, Sokol RJ, Balistreri WF, eds. *Liver Disease in Children*. 4th ed. Cambridge, United Kingdom: Cambridge University Press; 2014:111–139

Mieli-Vergani G, Vergani D. Autoimmune liver diseases in children—what is different from adulthood? *Best Pract Res Clin Gastroenterol*. 2011;25(6):783–795

Molleston JP, Fontana RJ, Lopez MJ, Kleiner DE, Gu J, Chalasani N; Drug-Induced Liver Injury Network. Characteristics of idiosyncratic drug-induced liver injury in children: results from the DILIN prospective study. *J Pediatr Gastroenterol Nutr*. 2011;53(2):182–189

Sturm E, Verkade HJ. Disorders of the intrahepatic bile ducts. In: Kleinman RE, Sanderson IR, Goulet O, Sherman PM, Mieli-Vergani G, Shneider BL, eds. *Walker's Pediatric Gastrointestinal Disease*. Vol 1. Hamilton, Ontario, Canada: BC Decker; 2008:803–815

Pancreatitis

Carmen Cuffari, MD

OVERVIEW

Pancreatitis is an uncommon disorder in children and adolescents that can be associated with significant morbidity and mortality. Recent studies have estimated the incidence of acute pancreatitis (AP) at about 1 in 10,000 children per year, which approaches the number reported in adults. About 25% to 30% of patients will experience acute recurrent episodes of pancreatitis secondary to genetic causes (eg, cystic fibrosis). It is not clear whether this increasing incidence represents a true rise in pediatric pancreatitis or improved awareness. The disease is classified as AP or chronic pancreatitis (CP), and occasionally is complicated by formation of a pseudocyst, a fibrous walled cavity within the body or tail of the pancreas that may communicate directly with the main pancreatic duct. Pseudocysts are generally filled with necrotic pancreatic tissue and digestive enzymes that might provide a nidus for infection and/or become large enough to displace the adjacent organs, including the common bile duct. In general, AP and CP in children are considered a disease continuum rather than 2 separate entities. A subset (up to 25%) of children with AP may develop severe pancreatic inflammation and necrosis, triggering a dangerous clinical condition termed *systemic inflammatory response syndrome* (SIRS) and multiorgan failure (shock, renal failure, pulmonary insufficiency).

CAUSES

Trauma and idiopathic disease are the most common causes of pancreatitis in children. Other less common causes of pancreatitis include congenital anomalies of the pancreaticobiliary system; systemic disorders, including lupus; drugs; viral infections; and metabolic disorders (**Box 15-1**). Pancreatitis also may result from direct injury to the acinar cells of the pancreas by means of viral infections, drugs, ischemia, and direct trauma. According to standard rigorous

Box 15-1. Causes of Childhood Pancreatitis

Idiopathic

Genetic mutations: chymotrypsin C (*CTRC*)

Trauma

Viral infection: mumps, rubella, coxsackie, HIV

Anomalies: pancreaticobiliary malunion, congenital anomalies of the pancreatobiliary junction, pancreas divisum, congenital sphincter of Oddi abnormality, choledochal cysts

Medications: azathioprine, tetracycline, L-asparaginase, valproic acid, corticosteroids, immunosuppressive agents, other agents

Metabolic abnormalities: hypertriglyceridemia, hyperglycemia

Hereditary pancreatitis: cystic fibrosis, serum protease inhibitor (*SPINK1*), protease inhibitors (*PRSS1*)

criteria (Evidence Level II-2), more than 40 drugs have been implicated in causing pancreatitis, many of which are used in children.

The inflammatory response may progress, depending on the extent of pancreatic injury, and result in vascular occlusion and ischemia, hemorrhage, and/or release of potent chemokines that can facilitate SIRS, disseminated intravascular coagulation (DIC), and multiorgan failure. Small pseudocysts generally resorb over time, whereas larger cysts often require surgical drainage, which can be facilitated by endoscopic retrograde cholangiopancreatography (ERCP) if the pseudocyst communicates with the main pancreatic duct or by transgastric stent placement.

SIGNS AND SYMPTOMS

The clinical signs of pancreatitis include severe epigastric abdominal pain, nausea, vomiting, and occasionally jaundice. Biochemical signs of pancreatitis include elevated serum amylase and lipase levels, and in cases of obstruction

of the common bile duct, hyperbilirubinemia and elevated levels of serum aminotransferases.

Abdominal pain and abdominal tenderness are the most common presenting symptoms in children with pancreatitis (>90% of affected children). Because the anatomical position of the duodenum is so intimately associated with the pancreas, inflammation extending from the pancreas to the duodenum can occur and lead to ileus, poor gastric emptying, and nausea and vomiting. In these children, eating may exacerbate the clinical symptoms.

Children with more severe forms of pancreatitis may require hospitalization, intravenous hydration, and hyperalimentation because of intractable nausea and vomiting. In addition, these patients often require intravenous forms of analgesia.

Fortunately, systemic complications are rare in children with AP. Acute hemorrhagic pancreatitis is an uncommon life-threatening complication of severe abdominal trauma. In these patients, complications of pancreatitis, including shock, DIC, and multiple organ dysfunction, as well as secondary infection may develop, with the mortality risk as high as 50%. The classic physical sign of hemorrhagic pancreatitis is discoloration of the flanks (ie, Grey Turner sign) or the periumbilical region (ie, Cullen sign) resulting from blood accumulation in the fascial planes of the abdomen.

EVALUATION

A diagnosis of pancreatitis typically rests on the presence of at least 2 of the following findings: typical abdominal pain, serum lipase/amylase levels higher than 3 times the upper limit of normal for age, and abnormal pancreatic imaging study findings consistent with inflammation (Evidence Level III), although some children with AP do not fulfill even 1 of these criteria.

Laboratory Studies

Serum amylase peaks about 48 hours after the onset of AP and typically remains elevated up to 4 days after the disease has subsided. Serum lipase elevations are more specific and slightly more sensitive than serum amylase elevations (Evidence Level II-2); in addition, they can remain elevated for up to 3 weeks after injury. Other laboratory tests, including those to detect coagulopathy, leukocytosis, hyperglycemia, hypocalcemia, hyperbilirubinemia, and serum aminotransferase abnormalities, can be performed and the results used in managing the disease and monitoring its clinical course.

Imaging Studies

Ultrasonography is the preferred radiological tool for evaluating the pancreas in children. Magnetic resonance (MR) cholangiopancreatography has essentially replaced computed tomography in evaluating CP and its complications in children. Endoscopic retrograde cholangiopancreatography is essential in evaluating pancreatic and biliary anomalies, and it can be useful in treating a number of complications associated with pancreatitis, as described earlier. Simple abdominal radiographs may be helpful in identifying sentinel loops of bowel in patients with significant nausea, vomiting, and abdominal distention; calcifications in children with CP; and gallstones in patients with biliary disease.

MANAGEMENT

Most cases of idiopathic AP in children resolve within 1 week of onset with pain control and intravenous hydration, and evidence shows that aggressive fluid therapy and early enteral feedings can shorten the illness course (Evidence Level II-1). Patients who develop large (>3 inches) pseudocysts may require surgical intervention (Evidence Level III). Most patients with CP complicated by scarring of the main pancreatic or hepatobiliary duct can develop an obstruction that requires surgical intervention.

Medical Management

Medical management aims at restoring normal metabolic function by means of rehydration and correction of acidosis and electrolyte imbalance. This can generally be accomplished without the need for parenteral hydration or nutrition. Acid suppression is helpful in preventing stress-induced gastritis and potential ulcer formation, as well as reducing duodenal acid exposure. Early and aggressive nutrition (oral, nasogastric, or nasojejunal) typically is safe in patients with AP and may promote more favorable outcomes, possibly by maintaining gut barrier function, preventing bacterial translocation, and lowering the risk of developing SIRS (Evidence Level II-2). In severe cases of AP, parenteral nutrition is often started within 5 days to prevent catabolism. In less severe forms of pancreatitis, a nasoduodenal feeding tube may be used to provide nutritional support by bypassing the duodenum entirely. Moreover, by bypassing the duodenum, the trophic stimulation of secretin and cholecystokinin is reduced. Acute pancreatitis should resolve in 2 to 7 days with supportive therapy. One study reported that a combination of early enteral nutrition (<48 hours) and aggressive fluid management (>1.5 to 2 times the patients' daily maintenance fluid requirements within the first 24 hours) decreased the length of hospital stay and complications (Evidence Level II).

In patients with chronic relapsing forms of pancreatitis, supportive therapy may need to be prolonged. Indeed, in patients with varying degrees of pancreatic insufficiency, a more protracted course of either nasoduodenal or parenteral nutritional therapy is often required. In the setting of chronic relapsing pancreatitis, pancreatic enzyme supplementation is often used. These supplements appear to optimize pancreatic rest in patients with AP and CP complicated by pancreatic insufficiency.

Surgical Management

In patients with chronic communicating pancreatic pseudocysts that fail to respond to supportive therapy, drainage stents may be inserted in the main pancreatic ducts via endoscopy. In patients with large, chronic noncommunicating pseudocysts, drainage catheters may be inserted endoscopically through the posterior wall of the stomach. Those with larger and more calcified pseudocysts may require cyst gastrostomy formation. Pseudocysts that are not accessible by means of conventional endoscopy may be drained by ultrasonography-guided or MR-guided percutaneous drainage. Surgical intervention, while rarely needed, is indicated for treatment of congenital anatomic defects, including pancreatic divisum. Moreover, ERCP can be helpful in diagnosing strictures of the main pancreatic duct and allowing for stent placement, thereby precluding the need for surgical intervention. Although the operative management of CP in children is controversial, distal pancreatectomy with Roux-en-Y pancreaticojejunostomy (ie, Duval procedure) or lateral pancreaticojejunostomy (ie, Puestow procedure) can be effective in refractory cases and in patients with intractable pain and narcotic dependency. In rare cases, total pancreatectomy and islet cell transplantation have been used to treat CP.

LONG-TERM CONSIDERATIONS

The long-term implications of CP in terms of its effect on patients' quality of life need to be underscored, especially in children. Most children with CP have underlying genetic abnormalities or poorly controlled metabolic disorders, including hyperlipidemia. In these patients, the adult perspective on management may be quite appropriate. Indeed, a complete pancreatectomy and islet cell implantation may be realistic long-term treatment options. More research is needed to evaluate methods of providing support to patients and parents that meets their needs.

SUGGESTED READING

Adamson WT, Hebra A, Thomas PB, Wagstaff P, Tagge EP, Othersen HB. Serum amylase and lipase alone are not cost-effective screening methods for pediatric pancreatic trauma. *J Pediatr Surg.* 2003;38(3):354–357

Adler DG, Baron TH, Davila RE, et al; Standards of Practice Committee of American Society for Gastrointestinal Endoscopy. ASGE guideline: the role of ERCP in diseases of the biliary tract and the pancreas. *Gastrointest Endosc.* 2005;62(1):1–8

Badalov N, Baradarian R, Iswara K, Li J, Steinberg W, Tenner S. Drug-induced acute pancreatitis: an evidence-based review. *Clin Gastroenterol Hepatol.* 2007;5(6):648–661

Bai HX, Lowe ME, Husain SZ. What have we learned about acute pancreatitis in children? *J Pediatr Gastroenterol Nutr.* 2011;52(3):262–270

Benifla M, Weizman Z. Acute pancreatitis in childhood: analysis of literature data. *J Clin Gastroenterol.* 2003;37(2):169–172

Kimble RM, Cohen R, Williams S. Successful endoscopic drainage of a posttraumatic pancreatic pseudocyst in a child. *J Pediatr Surg.* 1999;34(10):1518–1520

Morinville VD, Husain SZ, Bai H, et al; INSPPIRE Group. Definitions of pediatric pancreatitis and survey of present clinical practices. *J Pediatr Gastroenterol Nutr.* 2012;55(3):261–265

Nijs E, Callahan MJ, Taylor GA. Disorders of the pediatric pancreas: imaging features. *Pediatr Radiol.* 2005;35(4):358–373

Pohl JF, Uc A. Paediatric pancreatitis. *Curr Opin Gastroenterol.* 2015;31(5):380–386

Stringer MD, Davison SM, McClean P, et al. Multidisciplinary management of surgical disorders of the pancreas in childhood. *J Pediatr Gastroenterol Nutr.* 2005;40(3):363–367

Uc A, Fishman DS. Pancreatic disorders. *Pediatr Clin North Am.* 2017;64(3):685–706

Weckman L, Kylänpää ML, Puolakkainen P, Halttunen J. Endoscopic treatment of pancreatic pseudocysts. *Surg Endosc.* 2006;20(4):603–607

Peptic Ulcer Disease

Jyoti Sinha, MD; Patricia Eaton, DO; and Joel Rosh, MD

OVERVIEW

Peptic ulcer disease (PUD) is also referred to as gastric ulcer, gastritis, peptic ulcer, or acid-peptic disease. This disease may be divided into primary and secondary etiologies. Primary ulcers are more often chronic, duodenal in location, and complicated by fibrosis with fibrinopurulent debris overlying granulation tissue. Primary ulcers are unusual in children younger than 10 years and more prevalent in males. Secondary ulcers are usually acute, gastric in location, more common in children younger than 10 years, and do not demonstrate any sex preference. Secondary ulcers are commonly caused by physiologic stress or drug ingestion, and in general are not fibrotic. Most ulcers appear when there is a reduction of normal protective mechanisms such as local prostaglandins or an alteration of the gastric secretory function with increased hydrochloride acid production and pepsin activity. The hallmark of PUD is histologic evidence of a deep mucosal lesion with erosion of gastric or duodenal mucosa and disruption of the muscularis mucosa. The prevalence of PUD in pediatrics continues to be low and is much less common in children than in adults (Evidence Level III).

CLINICAL FEATURES/SIGNS AND SYMPTOMS

Clinical symptoms differ somewhat between age groups, can be nonspecific, and often overlap with functional gastrointestinal (GI) conditions (**Box 16-1**). The presence of warning signs and symptoms should shift the differential diagnosis from functional causes to the possibility of organic pathology such as PUD. In healthy infants, feeding difficulties and painful behavior are more commonly associated with overfeeding, milk protein intolerance, or colic. Infants and toddlers who present with failure to thrive, persistent vomiting, or hematemesis/melena should be referred promptly to a gastroenterologist for evaluation. Up to 25% of school-aged children will have functional GI complaints such as epigastric abdominal pain, anorexia, or nausea indicative of functional dyspepsia.

Box 16-1. Symptoms of Peptic Ulcer Disease

Infants and toddlers
- Feeding difficulties, vomiting, irritability, hematemesis, melena, failure to thrive

School-aged children
- Epigastric pain, nausea, vomiting, gastrointestinal bleeding, weight loss

Older children and adolescents
- Epigastric abdominal pain, abdominal fullness, dyspepsia, GI bleeding, weight loss

Other possible symptoms
- Iron deficiency anemia, anorexia, early satiety

However, weight loss, hematemesis, or melena raises the possibility of PUD or another organic pathology. In this age group, secondary ulcers are the predominate cause of PUD (**Box 16-2**). In older children and adolescents, both primary and secondary peptic ulcers occur more frequently than in younger children. Patients in this age group may report epigastric abdominal pain, fullness, or dyspepsia. The classic symptom of epigastric pain alleviated by food intake is present in only a minority of children. Complaints of abdominal pain are often poorly localized, may be periumbilical in location, and may cause nocturnal awakening. Ulcers induced by nonsteroidal anti-inflammatory drugs (NSAIDs) are characteristically asymptomatic until upper GI bleeding or perforation occurs. Rarely, PUD presents with an acute onset of constant, severe upper abdominal pain due to perforation, pancreatitis from a posterior penetrating ulcer, bright red blood per rectum due to brisk bleeding and a decreased intestinal transit time, or vomiting secondary to gastric outlet obstruction resulting from inflammation and fibrosis. With chronic disease, children may develop refractory iron deficiency anemia, weight loss, or anorexia.

Box 16-2. Differential Diagnosis of Dyspepsia

- Nonulcer functional dyspepsia
- Celiac disease
- Gastroesophageal reflux disease
- Cholecystitis
- Cholelithiasis
- Pancreatitis
- Lactose intolerance
- Inflammatory bowel disease

ETIOLOGIES

Peptic ulcer disease can be divided according to primary or secondary etiologies (**Box 16-3**). Primary ulcers are due to an infection with *Helicobacter pylori*, which accounts for more than 20% of duodenal ulcers in children. *Helicobacter pylori* is transmitted via the oral-oral or fecal-oral routes. Some children infected with *H pylori* develop histologic evidence of chronic active gastritis but are clinically asymptomatic. Although children may become infected at a very young age, clinical presentation is more common in adolescents. Other etiologies of primary PUD include hypersecretory states such as Zollinger-Ellison syndrome (gastrinoma), multiple endocrine neoplasia type I, antral G-cell hyperplasia, short bowel syndrome, cystic fibrosis, hyperparathyroidism, or systemic mastocytosis are rare in childhood.

Secondary ulcers are more common than primary ulcers and are caused by physiologic stress, drugs, or, rarely, hypersecretion. Multiple ulcers can develop in the stomach. Stress typically refers to patients with sepsis, shock, crush injuries, head trauma or an intracranial lesion (known as Cushing ulcer), severe burn injuries (Curling ulcer), or respiratory failure (especially when mechanical ventilation is needed). Lesions generally appear 3 to 6 days after the event. Aspirin and NSAIDs are typical causes of secondary PUD.

Box 16-3. Characteristics and Etiology of Peptic Ulcer Disease

Primary peptic ulcer disease	Secondary peptic ulcer disease

General characteristics

• Chronic	• Acute
• Duodenal	• Gastric
• More males than females	• Males equal females
• Children older than 10 y	• All ages
• Single lesions	• More common than primary disease
	• Multiple lesions

Etiologies

• *Helicobacter pylori* associated	• Physiologic stress (eg, sepsis, shock)
• Idiopathic	• Intracranial lesion (Cushing ulcer)
• Hypersecretory states:	• Severe burn injuries (Curling ulcer)
• Zollinger-Ellison syndrome	• Respiratory failure
• G-cell hyperplasia/hyperfunction	• Mechanical ventilation
• Systemic mastocytosis	• Crush injuries
• Cystic fibrosis	• Head trauma
• Short bowel syndrome	• Medications (eg, NSAIDs, valproic acid dexamethasone, chemotherapy, alcohol,
• Hyperparathyroidism	• Potassium chloride)
	• Crohn disease
	• Celiac disease
	• Chronic liver disease
	• Other severe systemic disease

Abbreviation: NSAID, nonsteroidal anti-inflammatory drug.

▼△▼△▼△▼△▼△▼△▼△▼   ▼△▼△▼△▼△▼△▼△▼△▼

EVALUATION

Evaluation of a patient with suspected PUD begins with a thorough history, including the initial onset and duration of symptoms with alleviating and exacerbating factors. The clinician should note predisposing risk factors with medical conditions along with a social and dietary history. In addition, the physician should obtain a family history of *H pylori* or gastritis. The physical examination focuses on the patient's growth rate. The oropharynx should be examined for enamel erosion, and dental caries indicates signs of reflux with persistent vomiting. Pale conjunctiva with tachycardia may suggest signs of blood loss or chronic systemic disease. The abdominal examination should focus on areas of tenderness and liver and spleen size. A rectal examination may identify a fissure or perianal disease.

The initial laboratory evaluation focuses on the presenting symptoms. A complete blood cell count identifies anemia and systemic inflammation. Blood in the GI tract can raise the blood urea nitrogen level, and a low albumin level may indicate a poor nutritional status, which is identified by a comprehensive metabolic profile (including electrolytes, liver chemistries). Inflammatory markers such as C-reactive protein and an erythrocyte sedimentation rate are helpful but not specific.

Noninvasive tests for *H pylori* include a urea breath test, which is best used as a marker of treatment success and infection eradication (Evidence Level III). A commercially available enzyme-linked immunosorbent assay (ELISA) for *H pylori* stool antigen is 98% sensitive and 99% specific and has a 98% positive predictive value. In contrast, serologic testing of blood, urine, or saliva generally is unreliable for clinical use, and the results do not correlate with the presence of active infection or demonstrate eradication of infection after therapy.

When to Refer for Upper Endoscopy

The gold standard diagnostic test is an esophagogastroduodenoscopy (EGD) or upper GI endoscopy to visualize the GI mucosa and obtain diagnostic biopsy tissues of the affected areas (Evidence Level III). Treatment also can be provided via an EGD in cases of an actively bleeding ulcer. Indications might include refractory anemia, refusal to eat, dysphagia, upper GI bleeding, odynophagia, constitutional symptoms, intractable vomiting, and pain despite acid-suppressant therapy. An accurate diagnosis of an initial infection with *H pylori* usually is established via EGD. The EGD with biopsy is the diagnostic test of choice to document mucosal disease as well as active infection with *H pylori*.

MANAGEMENT

The overall goals of PUD therapy are to heal the mucosa, treat the primary cause of the ulcer, relieve symptoms, and prevent complications and recurrence. As mentioned earlier, an EGD can be therapeutic in cases of active bleeding via hemostatic treatment including pressure, laser, thermal techniques, electrocoagulation, mechanical methods (clips, bands), or injection of epinephrine or saline. These techniques have an overall low complication rate, result in 75% to 90% control of active bleeding, and decrease the need for transfusions or emergency surgery. There is a 10% to 30% chance of rebleeding. Further, proton pump inhibitors (PPIs) are often used for acid suppression after endoscopic therapy (Evidence Level III).

The most familiar ulcer therapies are histamine-2 receptor antagonists (H2RAs) and PPIs, which are used for virtually all forms of the disease, including idiopathic ulcers and NSAID-induced disease (**Table 16-1**). Proton

Table 16-1. Recommended Treatment Regimens for Peptic Ulcer Disease

Medication	Recommended Dosage
Histamine-2 Receptor Antagonists	
Cimetidine	20–40 mg/kg/d divided 2–4 times daily
Ranitidine	4–10 mg/kg/d divided 2–3 times daily
Famotidine	1-2 mg/kg/d divided 2 times daily
Nizatidine	10 mg/kg/d divided 2 times daily
Proton Pump Inhibitors	
Omeprazole	<20 kg: 10 mg/d; >20 kg: 20 mg/d
Lansoprazole	<30 kg: 15 mg/d; >30 kg: 30 mg/d
Rabeprazole	Adult dose: 20 mg/d
Pantoprazole	Adult dose: 40 mg/d
Cytoprotective Agents	
Sucralfate	40–80 mg/kg/d divided into 4 doses/d

pump inhibitors are considered superior to H2RA blockers and do not exhibit the tachyphylaxis observed with H2RA blockers.

The consensus is that *H pylori* eradication should be reserved for cases associated with active PUD rather than just *H pylori* colonization (Evidence Level III). In light of the rising prevalence of antibiotic resistant strains, updated recommendations for diagnosis and treatment of *H pylori* were published in 2016. Antibiotic therapy may need to be tailored to susceptibility testing. When antibiotic susceptibility is not available, high-dose triple therapy with PPI, amoxicillin, and metronidazole or bismuth-based quadruple therapy is recommended. Treatment is administered for 14 days. In the event of treatment failure, a patient may require a course of rescue therapy with high-dose amoxicillin or bismuth-based quadruple therapy. Sequential 10-day therapy is equally effective with fully susceptible strains. Therapeutic success should be confirmed after 4 to 8 weeks with reliable noninvasive tests such as the stool antigen or urease breath test.

LONG-TERM CONSIDERATIONS

Although acid suppression is the mainstay of therapy for PUD, it can be associated with complications such as hospital-acquired pneumonia when used in the inpatient or intensive care unit setting, drug-drug interactions, and *Clostridium difficile* infection (noted especially with PPI therapy). The eradication of *H pylori* not only helps to resolve gastric and duodenal ulcers, but it also prevents recurrence. Cases of treatment failure are usually due to poor compliance with the complicated treatment regimens or resistance of the particular strain of bacteria present.

Complications of peptic ulcers include bleeding, perforation, and gastric outlet obstruction, all of which are rare in pediatrics.

SUGGESTED READING

Brown K, Lundborg P, Levinson J, Yang H. Incidence of peptic ulcer bleeding in the US pediatric population. *J Pediatr Gastroenterol Nutr.* 2012;54(6):733–736

Hua MC, Kong MS, Lai MW, Luo CC. Perforated peptic ulcer in children: a 20-year experience. *J Pediatr Gastroenterol Nutr.* 2007;45(1):71–74

Hyams JS, Di Lorenzo C, Saps M, Shulman RJ, Staiano A, van Tilburg M. Functional disorders: children and adolescents. *Gastroenterology.* 2016;150(6):1456–1468.e2

Jones NL, Koletzko S, Goodman K, et al; ESPGHAN, NASPGHAN. Joint ESPGHAN/NASPGHAN guidelines for the management of *Helicobacter pylori* in children and adolescents (update 2016). *J Pediatr Gastroenterol Nutr.* 2017;64(6):991–1003

Kalach N, Bontems P, Koletzko S, et al. Frequency and risk factors of gastric and duodenal ulcers or erosions in children: a prospective 1-month European multicenter study. *Eur J Gastroenterol Hepatol.* 2010;22(10):1174–1181

Malfertheiner P, Chan FK, McColl KE. Peptic ulcer disease. *Lancet.* 2009;374(9699):1449–1461

Oderda G, Mura S, Valori A, Brustia R. Idiopathic peptic ulcers in children. *J Pediatr Gastroenterol Nutr.* 2009;48(3):268–270

Rosen R, Vandenplas Y, Singendonk M, et al. Pediatric gastroesophageal reflux clinical practice guidelines: joint recommendations of the North American Society for Pediatric Gastroenterology, Hepatology, and Nutrition and the European Society for Pediatric Gastroenterology, Hepatology, and Nutrition. *J Pediatr Gastroenterol Nutr.* 2018;66(3):516–554

Tofil NM, Benner KW, Fuller MP, Winkler MK. Histamine 2 receptor antagonists vs intravenous proton pump inhibitors in a pediatric intensive care unit: a comparison of gastric pH. *J Crit Care.* 2008;23(3):416–421

Vomiting

John M. Olsson, MD

OVERVIEW

Vomiting is the forceful oral expulsion of gastric contents associated with contraction of the abdominal and chest wall musculature. Vomiting should be distinguished from regurgitation, which is the act by which food is brought back into the mouth without the abdominal and diaphragmatic muscular activity that characterizes vomiting. This review addresses the causes, evaluation, and management of vomiting in infants and children.

CAUSES AND DIFFERENTIAL DIAGNOSIS

A variety of conditions, both physical and psychological/behavioral, can cause vomiting in children. In addition to systemic and metabolic conditions, physical causes include conditions affecting the gastrointestinal, nervous, urinary, and endocrine systems (**Box 17-1**). Psychological/behavioral causes include rumination, bulimia, and psychogenic vomiting.

Separating causes of vomiting by age and the temporal pattern of vomiting is useful. Congenital and acquired obstructive lesions are more common causes of vomiting during infancy (**Table 17-1**), while vomiting caused by infectious, inflammatory, toxic, or endocrine issues are more common in older children and adolescents. Bilious vomiting suggests an intestinal obstruction distal to the ligament of Treitz (a peritoneal fold suspending the duodenojejunal flexure from the retroperitoneum) and warrants emergency evaluation and consultation with a pediatric surgeon) (**Box 17-2**). Bloody emesis can be caused by esophagitis/gastritis, peptic ulcer disease, Mallory-Weiss tears (ruptures of the mucous membrane where the esophagus meets the stomach), bleeding varices, or a Dieulafoy lesion (a large tortuous arteriole typically in the submucosal portion of the stomach wall that erodes and bleeds, but it can be present in any part of the gastrointestinal tract) (**Box 17-3**).

Box 17-1. Differential Diagnosis of Vomiting by System

Gastrointestinal

- Esophagus (stricture, web, ring, atresia, tracheo-esophageal fistula, achalasia, foreign body)
- Stomach (pyloric stenosis, web, duplication, peptic ulcer, gastroesophageal reflux)
- Intestine (duodenal atresia, malrotation, duplication, intussusceptions, volvulus, foreign body, bezoar, NEC)
- Colon (Hirschsprung disease, imperforate anus, foreign body, bezoar)
- Acute gastroenteritis
- *Helicobacter pylori* infection
- Parasitic infection (ascariasis, giardiasis)
- Appendicitis
- Milk/soy protein allergy
- Inflammatory bowel disease
- Pancreatitis
- Cholecystitis, cholelithiasis
- Hepatitis
- Peritonitis
- Trauma (duodenal hematoma)

Neurologic

- Tumor
- Cyst
- Hematoma
- Cerebral edema
- Hydrocephalus
- Pseudotumor cerebri
- Migraine headache
- Abdominal migraine
- Seizure
- Meningitis

Renal

- Obstructive uropathy (ureteropelvic junction obstruction, hydronephrosis, nephrolithiasis)
- Renal failure
- Glomerulonephritis

Box 17-1. Differential Diagnosis of Vomiting by System (*continued*)

Renal (*continued*)
- Urinary tract infection
- Renal tubular acidosis

Metabolic
- Galactosemia
- Hereditary fructosemia
- Amino acidopathy
- Organic acidopathy
- Urea cycle defect
- Fatty acid oxidation disorder
- Lactic acidosis
- Lysosomal storage disorder
- Peroxisomal disorder

Endocrine
- Diabetic ketoacidosis
- Adrenal insufficiency

Respiratory
- Pneumonia
- Sinusitis
- Pharyngitis

Miscellaneous
- Sepsis syndromes
- Pregnancy
- Rumination
- Bulimia
- Psychogenic
- Cyclic vomiting syndrome
- Overfeeding
- Medications/vitamin/drug toxicity
- Superior mesenteric artery syndrome
- Child abuse

Abbreviation: NEC, necrotizing enterocolitis.

From Chandran L, Chitkara M. Vomiting in children: reassurance, red flag, or referral? *Pediatr Rev.* 2008;29(6):183–192.

Table 17-1. Causes of Vomiting by Age and Temporal Pattern

Pattern	0–1 mo	1–12 mo	1–4 y	5–11 y	12–18 y
			Age		
Acute	• FPIES • Hirschsprung disease • Intestinal atresia • Meningitis • Pyloric stenosis • Sepsis	• Foreign body • FPIES • Gastroenteritis • Intussusception • UTI	• Foreign body • Gastroenteritis • Pharyngitis • Toxic ingestion • UTI • Constipation	• Appendicitis • Diabetic ketoacidosis • Pancreatitis	• Choledocholithiasis • Diabetic ketoacidosis • Drug overdose
Chronic	• Adrenal insufficiency • GERD • Hirschsprung disease • Intestinal atresia	• GERD	• Celiac disease • Eosinophilic esophagitis	• Celiac disease • Eosinophilic esophagitis • Gastritis +/– *Helicobacter pylori* • Gastroparesis • PUD	• Bezoar • CHS/marijuana use • Pregnancy

Cyclic	• Adrenal insufficiency
	• IEMs
	
	• Malrotation with
	  volvulus
		• Adrenal insufficiency
		• IEMs
		
		• Intussusception
		
		• Malrotation with
		  volvulus
			• Adrenal insufficiency
			• Constipation
				• Abdominal migraine
				• Cyclic vomiting syn-
				  drome
				• UPJ obstruction
					• Abdominal migraine
					• CHS/marijuana use
					
					• Cyclic vomiting
					  syndrome
					• Eating disorder
					
					• SMA syndrome
					• UPJ obstruction

Abbreviation: CHS, cannabinoid hyperemesis syndrome; FPIES, food protein-induced enterocolitis syndrome; GERD, gastroesophageal reflux disease; IEM, inborn errors of metabolism; PUD, peptic ulcer disease; SMA, superior mesenteric artery; UPJ, ureteropelvic junction; UTI, urinary tract infection.

From Shields TM, Lightdale JR. Vomiting in children. *Pediatr Rev.* 2018;39(7):342–358.

Box 17-2. Conditions That Can Cause Bilious Vomiting in Infancy

- Intestinal atresia and stenosis
- Malrotation with or without volvulus
- Meconium ileus
- Necrotizing enterocolitis
- Hirschsprung disease
- Inborn errors of metabolism
- Intussusception

EVALUATION

Determining hydration status and identifying the cause of the vomiting are 2 key clinical considerations in the evaluation and management of a child with vomiting.

The immediate concern is the child's hydration status and overall hemodynamic stability. Oral rehydration may be attempted for patients with mild or moderate dehydration secondary to acute gastroenteritis who are able to tolerate oral fluids (eg, electrolyte-containing solutions). For children with severe dehydration whose diagnosis is uncertain or who have acute gastroenteritis and in whom oral rehydration has failed, parenteral rehydration is required. In addition to restoring normal hydration, other supportive measures (ie, placement of a nasogastric tube when appropriate) should be considered before beginning a diagnostic evaluation.

Evaluating a child with vomiting begins with a thorough history and physical examination. A detailed history of vomiting includes its onset, frequency, duration, relationship to feeding, presence of bile, character of the vomiting, and determination of whether there is blood in the emesis. Additional details about feeding include changes in appetite, types of proteins being ingested, introduction of new foods, overall intake, formula preparation, and frequency of feedings. Signs such as fever, nausea, abdominal pain, diarrhea, rhinorrhea, otalgia, rash, cough, chest pain, or difficulty breathing may help identify causes. The medical history may suggest conditions that could predispose a child to gastrointestinal

Box 17-3. Differential Diagnosis of Hematemesis in Children

- Swallowed blood
  - Epistaxis
  - Breastfeeding
  - Dental work
  - Tonsillectomy
- Vitamin K deficiency in newborn
- Esophagitis
- Mallory-Weiss tear
- Hemorrhagic gastritis
- Severe systemic stress
  - Trauma
  - Surgery
- Peptic ulcer disease
- Submucosal masses
- Lipomas, stromal tumors, intestinal duplications
- Variceal bleeding, congestive gastropathy (associated with portal hypertension)
- Vascular malformations
- Angiodysplasia, hemangioma, Dieulafoy lesions
- Hemobilia
- Nonsteroidal anti-inflammatory drugs, radiation
- Systemic diseases—vasculitis (Henoch-Schönlein purpura), viral infection

obstructive disorders (eg, necrotizing enterocolitis or hemolytic-uremic syndrome with consequent intestinal stricture).

Additional considerations are a family history compatible with metabolic disease or conditions for which there is an increased familial prevalence (eg, Hirschsprung disease or pyloric stenosis). In addition to an assessment of hemodynamic status, the examination should be focused on the abdomen to note its appearance, such as distension. Bruising of the abdomen might suggest trauma,

▼▲▼▲▼▲▼▲▼▲▼▲▼▲▼▲   ▼▲▼▲▼▲▼▲▼▲▼▲▼▲▼

either as a result of an accident or child abuse. Auscultation of the abdomen before palpation may determine whether an ileus or a structural obstruction is present. In addition to noting the presence and location of any abdominal tenderness, the physician should palpate the abdomen for masses. Olive-shaped masses in the epigastric area suggest pyloric stenosis, and sausage-shaped masses in the right lower quadrant suggest intussusception.

When evaluating an infant for vomiting (**Figure 17-1**), the physician should determine whether it has an acute onset or an abrupt change in character, as opposed to vomiting that is chronic or recurrent in nature. In cases of acute vomiting, determining whether the emesis is bilious or nonbilious is key, with bilious emesis more often associated with an obstructive lesion warranting immediate evaluation. Workup for bilious emesis includes plain radiographs of the abdomen and an assessment for possible sepsis, another life-threatening cause of bilious emesis in infancy. Further workup will be dictated by the results of these studies. Consultation with a pediatric surgeon is warranted in cases in which prompt operative intervention may be required.

Infants with nonbilious vomiting may have an associated condition, such as otitis media or gastroenteritis, that does not require further evaluation. However, in infants with an uncertain diagnosis, additional workup might include an assessment of electrolyte levels, renal and hepatic function, and pancreatic enzymes, as well as metabolic studies (ie, ammonia, lactate, pyruvate) and a screen for sepsis. Radiographic studies may also be warranted if the history or physical examination findings suggest possible surgical diagnoses (eg, pyloric stenosis, intussusception). Continuing management depends on the results of these tests and ongoing clinical assessments.

For infants with chronic or persistent vomiting, distinguishing between gastroesophageal reflux, the most common cause of recurrent vomiting, and other causes is important. The vomiting observed in gastroesophageal reflux usually is not forceful, does not interfere with weight gain, and is a nuisance rather than a significant concern. However, more severe cases of gastroesophageal reflux and chronic vomiting that fail to meet the criteria for gastroesophageal reflux merit the same workup as that recommended for potential systemic causes in infants with acute nonbilious vomiting.

Attention to age-specific concerns also is necessary in the evaluation of a child or an adolescent (**Figure 17-2**). For example, an adolescent girl with vomiting may be pregnant, thereby prompting an appropriate history and a urine pregnancy test. The presentation should reveal details about the nature of the vomiting, frequency, associated symptoms, color, and presence or absence of blood in the emesis or stool. Also important is the patient's medical history, including surgeries, current medical conditions, and current medications, as

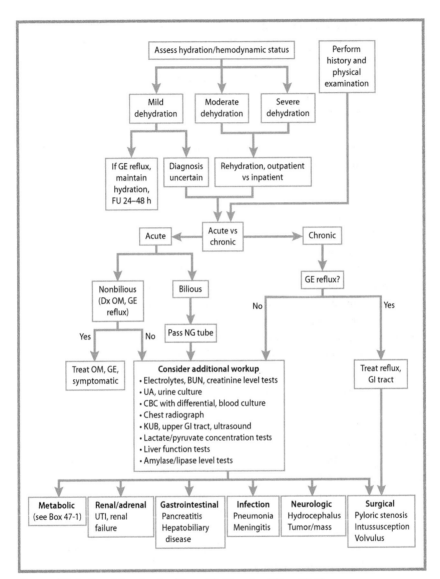

Figure 17-1. Vomiting in the First 12 Months After Birth

Abbreviations: BUN, blood urea nitrogen; CBC, complete blood cell count; Dx, diagnosis; FU, follow-up; GE, gastroesophageal; GI, gastrointestinal; KUB, kidney, ureter, and bladder; NG, nasogastric; OM, otitis media; UA, urinalysis; UTI, urinary tract infection; vs, versus.

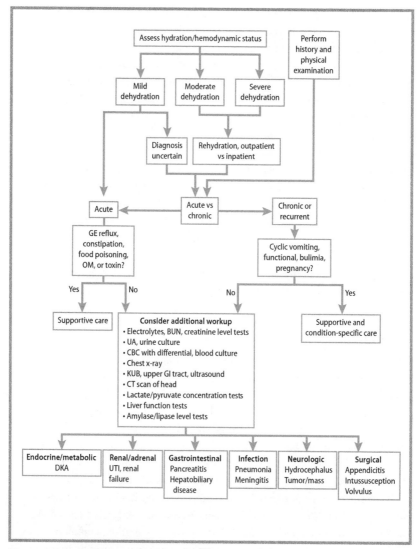

Figure 17-2. Vomiting Beyond Infancy

Abbreviations: BUN, blood urea nitrogen; CBC, complete blood cell count; CT, computed tomography; DKA, diabetic ketoacidosis; GE, gastroesophageal; KUB, kidney, ureter, and bladder; OM, otitis media; UA, urinalysis; UTI, urinary tract infection.

well as the family history, including inflammatory bowel disease and peptic ulcer disease, as these become more relevant in older children and adolescents.

The physician should distinguish acute from chronic presentations in a child or an adolescent with vomiting. Acute gastroenteritis is the most common cause of acute vomiting in children and adolescents. Diarrhea is usually associated with vomiting in cases of gastroenteritis. When vomiting is the only presenting symptom, the physician must carefully consider alternative diagnoses. Severe constipation, toxic ingestions, food poisoning, streptococcal throat infection, and otitis media are other causes of vomiting that are identifiable by history and physical examination findings. If, however, the patient does not meet the clinical criteria for these diagnoses or the vomiting is chronic or lasts longer than is consistent with acute gastroenteritis, the differential diagnosis should be expanded. In such cases, electrolyte levels, renal and liver function tests, urinalysis and urine culture, metabolic studies (eg, venous pH, glucose, ketones), and pancreatic enzymes should be considered.

Imaging studies of the head, chest, and abdomen may be required depending on the patient's examination findings and status.

MANAGEMENT

Treatment is directed at correcting the underlying cause of vomiting and restoring a normal hydration status (Evidence Level III). If the disease is mild and no specific etiology is identified, the patient should be treated symptomatically with fluids to maintain hydration (Evidence Level I). In general, antiemetic medications, which are often used in adults, should be avoided in children because of the serious potential adverse effects seen with phenothiazines and metoclopramide in this age group. A recent Cochrane review provided strong evidence (Evidence Level I) for ondansetron treatment in children and adolescents with vomiting that is associated with acute gastroenteritis in the emergency department. Children treated with ondansetron were less likely to be admitted to the hospital, less likely to require intravenous rehydration, and more likely to stop vomiting. Antiemetic treatment with ondansetron should be limited to management of vomiting caused by acute gastroenteritis, although ondansetron has been shown to reduce vomiting in children receiving chemotherapy and radiation therapy (Evidence Level I), as well as in those who have postoperative nausea and vomiting (Evidence Level I). Evidence supporting its benefit on a continuing outpatient basis is lacking, so a patient who is vomiting for more than 2 to 3 days after an initial visit should be reexamined.

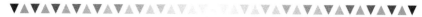

SUGGESTED READING

Allen K. The vomiting child—what to do and when to consult. *Aust Fam Physician*. 2007;36(9): 684–687

Chandran L, Chitkara M. Vomiting in children: reassurance, red flag, or referral? *Pediatr Rev*. 2008; 29(6):183–192

DeCamp LR, Byerley JS, Doshi N, Steiner MJ. Use of antiemetic agents in acute gastroenteritis: a systematic review and meta-analysis. *Arch Pediatr Adolesc Med*. 2008;162(9):858–865

Fedorowicz Z, Jagannath VA, Carter B. Antiemetics for reducing vomiting related to acute gastro-enteritis in children and adolescents. *Cochrane Database Syst Rev*. 2011;9:CD005506

Shields TM, Lightdale JR. Vomiting in children. *Pediatr Rev*. 2018;39(7):342–358

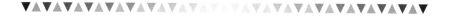

Index

Page numbers followed by an *f*, a *t*, or a *b* denote a figure, a table, or a box, respectively.

▼▲▼▲▼▲▼▲▼▲▼▲▼▲▼▲   ▲▼▲▼▲▼▲▼▲▼▲▼▲▼